D1756498

Topics in Pharmacy
Volume 2
Routes of Drug Administration

THEATRE
GRANTHAM

Routes of
Drug Administration

Edited by

A. T. Florence PhD, DSc, FRSC, FRSE, FRPharmS

The School of Pharmacy,
University of London,
London, UK

and

E. G. Salole BSc, PhD, MRPharmS

Department of Pharmacy,
University of Strathclyde,
Glasgow, UK

WRIGHT

London   Boston   Singapore   Sydney   Toronto   Wellington

Wright
is an imprint of Butterworth Scientific

 PART OF REED INTERNATIONAL P.L.C.

First published 1990

© Butterworth & Co. (Publishers) Ltd, 1990

British Library Cataloguing in Publication Data

Routes of drug administration.
1. Medicine. Drug therapy
I. Florence, A. T. (Alexander Taylor)   II. Salole, E. G.
(Eugene G)   III. Series
615.6

ISBN 0-7236-0922-5

Library of Congress Cataloging-in-Publication Data

Routes of drug administration/edited by A. T. Florence
and E. G. Salole.
    p. cm.—(Topics in pharmacy; v. 2)
    Includes bibliographical references.
    ISBN 0-7236-0922-5
    1. Drugs—Administration.   I. Florence, A. T.
(Alexander Taylor)   II. Salole, E. G.   III. Series.
    [DNLM: 1. Drug Administration Routes.
QV 785 R869]
RM147.R68   1990
615'.6—dc20

Composition by Genesis Typesetting, Laser Quay, Rochester, Kent
Printed and bound in England by Page Bros. Ltd, Norwich, Norfolk

Series preface

There is, in our view, an important need to draw the attention of both students and practitioners concerned with drug therapy to recent and continuing developments in the pharmaceutical sciences. The purpose of the *Topics in Pharmacy* series is to fulfil this need by providing up-to-date, concise, readable accounts of current aspects of pharmacy – with particular emphasis on those aspects of the pharmaceutical sciences related to clinical practice. In this endeavour we have been fortunate in securing the collaboration of academics and practitioners recognized as experts in the subjects of their contributions.

Each volume in the series has a theme, and each constituent chapter provides a concise account of a particular area; the accounts are intended to be introductions to a topic rather than comprehensive and complete reviews, and hence, wherever possible, each chapter is appended with a short bibliography for further study.

The series is aimed at a readership comprising senior undergraduate and postgraduate students in pharmacy, medicine, nursing and allied health sciences, and practitioners in these fields. However, it is our hope that the series will also be generally useful to other professionals concerned with the preparation and administration of medicines and the monitoring of drug therapy.

Alexander T. Florence, London
Eugene G. Salole, Glasgow

Preface

Oral administration, the commonest and most convenient route for delivery of drugs to the systemic circulation, is not always the most suitable, for example in the elderly or the seriously ill. Indeed, the oral route may not be an option for systemic action of a range of drugs which are poorly absorbed from the gastrointestinal tract, through inappropriate intrinsic physical properties, degradation or metabolism. This volume, the second in the *Topics in Pharmacy* series, describes a number of parenteral routes of administration, some of which, such as the transdermal route, are increasingly finding favour as viable alternatives to the enteral route. Others such as the nasal and buccal routes will possibly find a place in therapy with a more limited group of drugs.

The theme of Volume 1 of this series, the interaction of formulations with the biological milieu, is continued in this volume, as individual chapters review the anatomy and physiology of administration sites, the formulation and design of delivery systems and other relevant aspects of biopharmaceutics. Dosage form behaviour *in vivo* has to be taken into account in the design of the delivery system. The success or failure of a system can depend on the anatomy of the route and the tailoring of the formulation to it. Nowhere is this better illustrated than in pulmonary delivery. This route and the nasal, buccal and transdermal routes of administration for systemic delivery are considered in this volume, as are a number of systems for more localized therapy with antibiotics.

We are indebted to Professor Lawrence Danziger, Dr Stephen Farr, Professor Ian Kellaway, Dr Philip Lamey, Dr Michael Lewis, Dr Graham Parr, Dr Alan Rogerson, Professor Jill Shwed, Dr Glyn Taylor and Dr Kenneth Walters for their sustained interest and contributions to this book.

Alexander T. Florence, London
Eugene G. Salole, Glasgow

Contributors

L. H. Danziger, PharmD
Assistant Professor of Pharmacy Practice, The University of
Illinois at Chicago, USA

S. J. Farr, BSc, PhD, MRPharmS
Lecturer in Pharmaceutics, Welsh School of Pharmacy,
University of Wales College of Cardiff, Cardiff, UK

I. W. Kellaway, BPharm, PhD, MRPharmS
Professor of Pharmaceutics, Welsh School of Pharmacy,
University of Wales College of Cardiff, Cardiff, UK

P.-J. Lamey, BSc, BDS, MBChB, DDS, FDS
Senior Lecturer and Honorary Consultant in Oral Medicine &
Pathology, University of Glasgow, Glasgow, UK; Visiting
Professor of Stomatology, Baylor College of Dentistry, Dallas,
Texas, USA

M. A. O. Lewis, BDS, PhD, FDS
Lecturer in Oral Medicine and Pathology, University of
Glasgow, Glasgow, UK

G. D. Parr, BSc, PhD, MRPharmS
Group Head, Pharmaceutical Development, Reckitt & Colman
Products Ltd, Hull, UK

A. Rogerson, BSc, PhD, MRPharmS
Senior Section Manager, Prescription Product Development,
Reckitt & Colman Products Ltd, Hull, UK

J. A. Shwed, PharmD
Assistant Professor of Hospital Pharmacy Practice and
Administration, Medical University of South Carolina,
Charleston, USA

G. Taylor, BSc, PhD, MRPharmS
Lecturer in Pharmaceutics, Welsh School of Pharmacy,
University of Wales College of Cardiff, Cardiff, UK

K. A. Walters, PhD
Director of Research & Development, Pharmaserve Ltd,
Swinton, Manchester, UK

Contents

1

Nasal drug delivery

A. Rogerson and G. D. Parr

Introduction

In most mammals the major function of the nose is as an olfactory organ, and sense of smell has a vital role in activities as diverse as hunting, and recognizing young. In man, although its function is no longer vital to survival, the importance of the nose should not be underestimated: in the seventeenth century Blaise Pascal noted that 'if Cleopatra's nose had been shorter, the whole history of the world would have been different'!

In its simplest form the nose is a passage through which air must pass *en route* to the lungs, and thus the modification of inspired air is probably its most important function in man. The nose consists of three distinguishable regions (Figures 1.1 and 1.2). The nostrils act to gather and direct air. Behind the nostrils lies the region which contains the convoluted turbinates and the nasal epithelium. This region leads into the nasopharynx, where the septum (which divides the nasal cavity into two halves) ends and the cavity becomes one. From the nostrils to the nasopharynx is generally a distance of *c.* 12–15 cm. When air is inspired it travels in an approximately parabolic pattern from the nostrils, upwards through the middle meatus, generally bypassing the turbinates, then downwards again through the nasopharynx (Figure 1.1). To pass into the nasal cavity, air must first be inspired with sufficient linear velocity to pass through the constriction of the nasal valve just beyond the nostrils.

Within the central region of the nasal cavity lie the ciliated nasal epithelial cells. This region presents a barrier to the absorption of drugs and contaminants that is relatively thin (and unkeratinized, despite its continuity with the exterior) and well perfused by nasal blood vessels. However, any drug substance applied nasally would rarely come into prolonged intimate contact with the epithelial cell surface owing to the presence of mucus glands and goblet cells (Figure 1.3). Mucus is a glycoprotein which is stored within goblet cells in its dehydrated form (containing *c.* 5% water), and is then hydrated as it

1

2

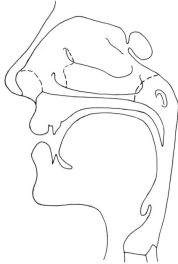

Figure 1.1 A side view of the upper respiratory tract. In the diagram, the left-hand dashed line (just behind the nostrils) indicates the region of the nasal valve; the intermediate dashed line indicates the approximate region of the ciliated epithelial mucosa, which ends near the termination of the nasal septum at the pharynx (indicated by the right-hand dashed line)

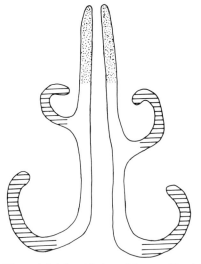

Figure 1.2 A frontal view of the nasal tract. The upper olfactory region (stippled area) is generally free from inspired air. The clear areas either side of the central nasal septum indicate the zone which is lined with absorptive epithelial cells and most accessible to inspired air

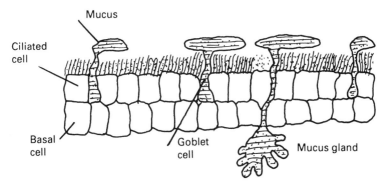

Figure 1.3 Schematic representation of ciliated epithelium overlaid with discontinuous mucus and periciliary fluid. The cilia beat in periciliary fluid, with a velocity gradient which is greatest at their apex

is released, swelling rapidly to form a layer (which may or may not be continuous) on top of the ciliated epithelial cells. Thus, mucus, which contains 95% water when fully hydrated, is responsible for the protection of the nasal epithelium, as it normally prevents intimate contact of epithelial cells with inspired material. The upper layers of mucus are propelled by the tips of the beating cilia, so that any airborne contaminants that may become associated with the periciliary fluid are forced backwards into the nasopharynx and swallowed. Clearance from the nasal cavity by means of ciliary expulsion proceeds at a rate of c. 5–6 mm/min. However, if contaminants penetrate the mucus layer, or if mucus is absent in certain regions, then it becomes almost impossible for the cilia to clear material from the nasal cavity. The degree of continuity of the mucus layer within the nasal cavity is not known, although particles appear to be transported at a relatively uniform rate irrespective of their size, density or composition. In addition, the viscosity of mucus is believed not to affect this expulsion of material, and poor transport is probably a consequence of inadequate cilia density, poor beating coordination or alterations in the composition of mucus[1].

It is impossible to avoid inspiration of contaminating particles. The atmosphere contains materials that range from metallurgical dusts and fumes (some particles of which may be c. 1 nm in diameter), tobacco smoke, bacteria and viruses (0.1–10 μm) to dusts and sand (≤ 1 mm diameter). Thus, many disorders, which may include both local irritation and inflammation (e.g.

allergic rhinitis), and systemic bacterial and viral infections, are mediated by nasal inspiration of atmospheric contaminants.

Nasally administered dosage forms generally deliver most of the drug to the ciliated region and, consequently, residence time is unlikely to be longer than a few minutes. The expulsion of drug by the cilia may be reduced (at least to some extent) by utilizing formulations that contain mucoadhesive materials (e.g. polyacrylic acid). These attach themselves to the mucus layer allowing a relatively long and intimate contact with the epithelial cell surface. Generally, pharmaceutical nasal dosage forms do not rely on adhesion to the mucus layer.

For a given aerosol the most important criteria in determining the site of deposition are particle diameter and size distribution, and the velocity of the aerosol particles[2]. The three most common mechanisms of deposition are shown in Figure 1.4.

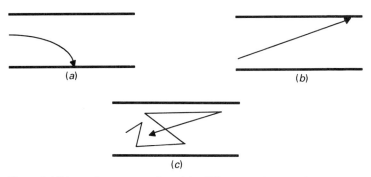

Figure 1.4 Schematic representation of the different mechanisms for particle deposition within the nasal cavity: *a*, gravity; *b*, inertial impaction; *c*, Brownian movement

Inspired particles are prone to the downward pull of gravity: those that are particularly large and dense do not penetrate far into the nasal cavity. Impaction is most likely to take place when an airstream carrying an aerosol particle rapidly changes direction: therefore, because of the shape of the nasal cavity, it is unlikely that a large number of particles will be deposited in the deeper regions. Other criteria, such as random diffusion and electrical effects, are mainly of only theoretical interest.

The presence of the nasal valve, and the sharp bend in the pathway taken by inspired air just beyond it, are responsible for the deposition of many aerosol particles within the anterior nasal region, where very little absorption takes place. In addition, poorly soluble drug particles or non-adhesive carrier systems that are delivered to the epithelial surface will be cleared by the cilia. Thus, as will be discussed later, the design of both the dosage solution and delivery device are critically important, as the physical characteristics of the presentation can profoundly affect the deposition, and subsequent efficacy, of the drug.

It is apparent that, even under ideal conditions, the choice of appropriate dosage form for nasal delivery is a multifaceted issue. When pathological conditions (which can profoundly alter the nasal cavity) exist, the problem becomes considerably more complex. Even in the absence of disease states, the intimate contact of the nasal mucosa with the atmosphere makes it susceptible to variations in temperature and humidity, and trauma to the nasal epithelium is apparently more common in the world's colder regions[3].

In terms of potential drug absorption across epithelial cells, the nasal cavity is not markedly different from the gastrointestinal (GI) tract. However, the surface area available for absorption is comparatively very small (the GI tract is often said to have a surface area equivalent to that of a tennis court – on the same scale the nasal cavity would be equivalent to one of the holes in the net!) and, in addition, the ciliated epithelial cells allow only short residence times for any drugs applied. As is discussed later, many methods of overcoming these problems have been investigated, including altering epithelial permeability and adhering dosage forms to mucus. Additionally, because of the absence of intestinal acid and degradative enzymes, the nasal route has been considered for non-oral delivery of labile drug molecules such as insulin[4] and LHRH analogues[5].

Assessment of nasal absorption

Generally, it is neither practical nor economically viable to test nasal preparations routinely in human subjects: the spiralling costs of clinical trials dictate that only a few formulations may be tested in this manner. Thus, it is essential that alternative methods of screening potential drugs and formulations are utilized. The use of model systems usually tends to be a compromise between cost, availability of the appropriate animal species and the degree of correlation with clinical results.

In order to determine whether a drug molecule is likely to be absorbed, or to assess the effects of penetration enhancers, probably the most accessible and least expensive model is the rat. Most model systems using this animal are variations on the procedure by Hirai *et al.* [6]. Rats are anaesthetized and an incision made in the neck, allowing the trachea to be exposed and cannulated. An incision is then made into the oesophagus, a polythene tube inserted, and the oesophagus sealed with adhesive to prevent drainage of drug solution from the nasal cavity (Figure 1.5). When the rat has been prepared in this manner two options are available. Without further modification, solutions of drug (penetration enhancer may also be included) may be introduced into the nasal cavity by means of the polythene tube, the tube closed and regular blood samples withdrawn and assayed for absorbed drug. This procedure has the potential advantage of providing pharmacokinetic information, which can often be useful before more extensive work in humans. However, for more fundamental research a further modification of the system may be more appropriate: the rat is inverted and tipped, so that drug solution is allowed to drain forwards from the nasal cavity, and is subsequently recycled (by means of a peristaltic pump), ensuring prolonged exposure of

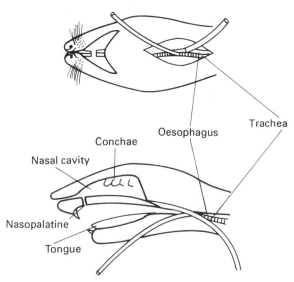

Figure 1.5 The top and side views of rats that have been surgically treated to facilitate administration of nasal solutions. (From reference 7)

mucosa to drug (Figure 1.6). Assay of solutions from experiments of this nature does not involve the extraction of drug from biological fluids, and therefore may be relatively rapid and simple. However, a potential problem is that the large volume of solution required compromises assay sensitivity. It is generally accepted that the former model (the so-called *in vivo* model) is superior, as it is more representative of the application of nasal drops or spray in clinical practice; in addition, the absorption profiles from this model tend to be superior for hydrophilic, lipophilic and peptide drugs[6]. The *in vivo* model has been used extensively to assess the nasal absorption of drugs such as salicylates[6], propranolol[9], cromoglycate[10], enkephalins[11], LHRH analogues[12] and insulin[13]. Absorption models, utilizing larger animals, have also been reported. Hussain[14] investigated the nasal absorption of propranolol in anaesthetized rats and dogs. In dogs, surgery was kept to a minimum and the nasal solution was simply introduced by means of a micropipette, with blood samples being withdrawn

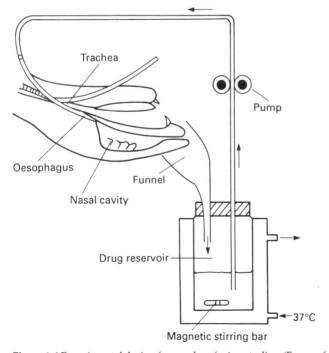

Figure 1.6 Experimental design for nasal perfusion studies. (From reference 8)

from the cubital vein. A larger animal model, sheep, has been used to study nasally administered insulin[4]. It was not clear whether the animals had been anaesthetized; however, in the presence of sodium taurodihydrofucidate, insulin was rapidly absorbed and reached peak levels in <15 min. The kinetics of absorption were very reproducible, and apparently similar to those reported for other species[13] and man[15].

Other species have been studied as potential animal models for nasal absorption. Anik et al. [5] investigated the absorption of a nasally administered LHRH analogue to anaesthetized rhesus monkeys: in general, the drug was poorly absorbed and bioavailability figures were of the order of 1%. Johnson et al. [16] compared the relative effects of human leucocyte interferon in man and chimpanzees. However, as was also the case for kinetics in dogs[14], these results indicated that there was little significance in the differences between absorption in rats and in larger animal models. Thus, from the point of view of convenience and expense, there would appear to be little reason for utilizing larger animals in primarily investigational work.

Many studies have been undertaken in human volunteers. Because blood sampling can often be extremely time-consuming, particularly at the analytical stage, non-invasive techniques have been developed, offering the advantages of greater frequency of testing and less discomfort to subjects. Hardy et al. [17] reported a study in which nasal sprays and drops of human serum albumin which had been labelled with gamma-emitting Tc^{99m} were administered, and the patterns of deposition of labelled material within the nasal cavity assessed with a gamma camera (Figure 1.7). The results suggested that drops provided better delivery over the whole surface area and generally confirmed the findings of Aoki and Crawley[18] who utilized a similar, although less sophisticated, experimental technique. The capacity of various drug carrier systems to retard the rate of nasal clearance was investigated in man using gamma scintigraphy[19]. This carrier effect is discussed in detail in a later section (page 19).

An alternative to non-invasive gamma scintigraphy is the direct measurement of serum drug levels. This approach has been employed for many drugs, including propranolol[14], oestrogen[20], oxytocin[21] and insulin[22]. Advantages of this type of assessment include the acquisition of pharmacokinetic data without extrapolation from other species. In addition to the assessment of serum drug levels, models utilizing man also offer the potential for assessment of biological effect, e.g. the

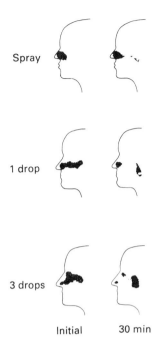

Figure 1.7 Sites of deposition and patterns of clearance within the nasal cavity following administration of radio-labelled nasal spray and drops. (From reference 17)

psychotropic effects of cocaine[23], dry mouth from hyoscine[24], uterine contractions from oxytocin[25] and improved exercise tolerance with glyceryl trinitrate[26].

In a logical sequence of progression it would be reasonable first to determine the rate and extent of absorption of a drug using an animal model, subsequently to optimize the formulation, then to dose human volunteers to obtain such information as the pharmacokinetic profile of the drug. Thus, although various animal models have been utilized, their results must not be taken in isolation. It is essential that before any animal model is used routinely its correlation with man is demonstrated.

In an attempt to determine the feasibility of dosing by the nasal route, Su and Campanale[7] reported the use of a 'false nose' (Figure 1.8) through which they administered solutions of drugs in the form of drops, nebulizers, automated pumps and pressurized aerosols. Their results suggested that for a pressurized aerosol system the ideal means of delivery is two puffs per nostril, with one puff in the upper direction and one in the lower.

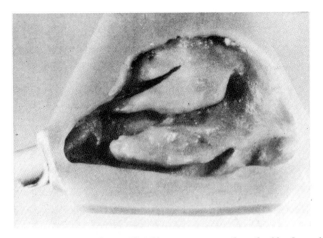

Figure 1.8 A cast of an artificial human nose, as described by Su and Campanale. The distribution of administered solution may be determined visually. (From reference 7)

Any conclusions about the potential usefulness of nasal administration of a drug are only as reliable as the methods of assessment. Great care must be taken in the choice of model, etc., and, as far as possible, correlation with man should be ensured [27].

Drug absorption across the nasal mucosa

As in the case of the GI tract, it is generally recognized that the absorption of a drug across the nasal mucosa is a function of its physicochemical properties, particularly its partition coefficient. In order to be absorbed a drug generally must partition from solution into the mucosal cell layers, across the cell layers and into the systemic circulation. Thus, a balance between water solubility and lipid solubility is necessary for optimal absorption characteristics. In practice this generalization does not always apply, as Hirai and colleagues observed [6]. They reported significant absorption of salicylic acid even at high pH, suggesting that the drug crossed the nasal mucosa even in its ionized state, and they concluded that nasal absorption is dictated not only by the nature of the undissociated molecule, but also by its lipid solubility, binding to mucosa and subsequent absorption of the ionized species.

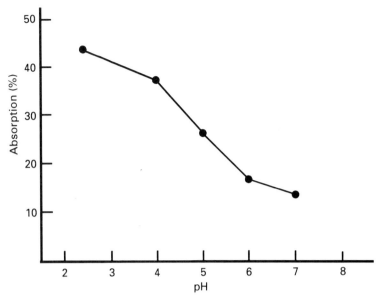

Figure 1.9 The percentage of benzoic acid absorbed in 60 min in the rat nasal perfusion model as a function of pH of the nasal perfusion solution. (From reference 8)

The effect of pH and partition coefficient on nasal absorption of benzoic acid was studied in the rat model *in vitro* by Hussain *et al.* [8]. Benzoic acid has a pK_a of 4.20 and, as expected, the extent of absorption was inversely related to pH (Figure 1.9). However, even at pH 7.2, when the drug is about 99.9% ionized, there was significant (13%) nasal absorption. Calculation of absorption rate constants led to the conclusion that undissociated drug was absorbed about four times faster than the ionized acid.

Lipid-soluble drugs

The absorption of lipophilic drugs is often rate-limited by their inability to partition out of epithelial cell layers and into the systemic circulation. However, the nasal mucosa is very thin, with a well-developed network of blood vessels [6], and therefore the physical barrier to systemic absorption is much less marked. Furthermore, as has been demonstrated for epithelial cell monolayers, many lipophilic drugs may be absorbed by an extracellular or paracellular pathway [28].

Oral treatment with propranolol, an adrenergic β-blocker, gives rise to variable plasma levels which become more reproducible on repeated dosing, but oral bioavailability can be as low as 16% [29]. This is attributed to extensive drug metabolism during absorption and on first pass through the liver. Investigation of intranasal delivery of propranolol to dogs revealed that plasma profiles very similar to those obtained after intravenous (i.v.) administration could be obtained [9, 14], and that the bioavailability of nasal propranolol was essentially 100% (Figure 1.10). The bioavailability of propranolol from a 2% methylcellulose nasal gel and a propranolol hydrochloride oral tablet were compared in human subjects: the nasal gel and an i.v. infusion gave identical results, whereas the tablet yielded bioavailability values of *c.* 25% [30]. Although these results show considerable promise, the probability of a nasal formulation of propranolol being marketed is very low, for two reasons:

1. First-pass metabolism is a problem for single-dose treatment, but the dose can often be increased to account for this and, in this particular case, dosage increases are generally not required as propranolol produces biologically active metabolites;

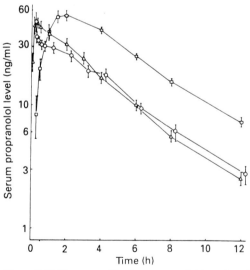

Figure 1.10 Plasma profiles for propranolol in male volunteers following administration of 10 mg intranasally (△), 10 mg intravenously (○) and 80 mg orally (□) (mean ± SD; $n = 6$). (From reference 30)

2. Therapy with propranolol is usually chronic, so the effect of the drug on the nasal mucosa must be considered – a nose drop solution containing as little as 0.1% propranolol has been shown to arrest irreversibly the ciliary capacity of human adenoid tissue after only 20 min exposure [31].

Despite its obvious shortcomings as a route for chronic therapy, there is a possible use for nasal propranolol in the acute treatment of myocardial infarction during first aid. In that case the effects of the drug on the cilia would be of little consequence if a life-threatening condition were being treated adequately.

Buprenorphine is an opiate analgesic that displays a low oral bioavailability (5%) owing to inactivation by enzymes in the gut wall and extensive first-pass metabolism in the liver [32]. The problem of low oral bioavailability may be overcome (to a degree) by utilizing the sublingual route of administration, but while first-pass metabolism is reduced, the onset of maximum effect is delayed to 2–3 h. In a rat model, Hussain and colleagues [33] have shown that the drug is absorbed rapidly and reproducibly by the nasal route (Figure 1.11). These data

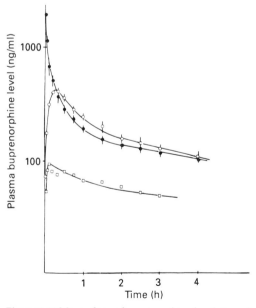

Figure 1.11 Mean plasma buprenorphine levels in male rats following administration of 135 μg nasally (○), intravenously (●) and intraduodenally (□) (mean ± SEM; $n = 4$). (From reference 33)

confirm that buprenorphine is extensively absorbed nasally, with peak levels at around 30 min after administration, after which the kinetics are identical to an i.v. dose. As shown in Table 1.1, the relative bioavailability of nasal buprenorphine compares very favourably with other non-oral routes of administration in rats[32].

Table 1.1 Bioavailability of buprenorphine administered to rats by various routes (from reference 32)

Route	Relative bioavailability (%)
Nasal	95
Rectal	54
Sublingual	13
Intraduodenal	10

In order to utilize naturally occurring ovarian hormones as contraceptive agents, they must be available in high concentration to exert their effects centrally. As they undergo extensive first-pass metabolism following oral administration, the doses required are often sufficiently large to induce extensive side-effects[34]. There would appear to be a strong case for use of the nasal route for administration of endogenous and synthetic steroids. Anand Kumar and colleagues[34] demonstrated that a greater concentration of oestradiol and progesterone was observed in the CSF following treatment with a nasal spray than with i.v. injection; in addition, simultaneous hormone levels in the peripheral tissues were lower. They concluded that there may be two pathways by which these steroids could reach the brain: either via the nasal epithelium or via the olfactory neurones. In another experiment, administration to monkeys of 2 µg progesterone in a nasal spray was successful in suppressing ovulation, but on raising the dose to 10–300 µg ovulation was not affected[35], indicating that nasal administration is a method of selecting the inhibitory or facilitatory effects of progesterone.

Water-soluble drugs

The nasal epithelium is very thin and well perfused by blood vessels, and the mucosal surface is constantly wetted by secretions[6]. Thus, the aqueous solubility of a drug is an important factor in determining its nasal absorption. This was demonstrated by Tonndorf and coworkers[24], who compared the relative effectiveness of nasal atropine and hyoscine by assessing their capacity to arrest salivary secretion and concluded that 0.65 mg hyoscine (which is *c.* 40 times more soluble in water) was equivalent to 2 mg atropine. These results, and others documenting extensive absorption of fully ionized benzoic acid[8], suggest that a high partition coefficient may not be the only prerequisite for nasal absorption. Further evidence of this nature has been reported by Fisher and colleagues[10]. They investigated the nasal absorption of sodium cromoglycate, a dibasic drug with negligible lipophilicity in the ionized state, and detected plasma levels equivalent to >70% of the administered dose. Clearly, all these data suggest that an alternative route of absorption is present, and it has been suggested that there is significant absorption through aqueous pores (or channels) within the nasal mucosa[6, 36]. Further evidence for the 'aqueous pores' theory is abundant, as many small highly hydrophilic molecules have been investigated for delivery by the nasal route.

Probably the drug most immediately associated with the nasal route is cocaine – a CNS stimulant and local anaesthetic. Indeed, such is the effectiveness of the nasal route that an intense 'high' is generally produced in <5 min; plasma levels peak at around 60 min and decrease gradually for up to 5 h[23]. The long duration of action is thought to be partly related to the drug's local vasoconstrictive action.

Hydralazine is a potent antihypertensive agent which, like propranolol, is routinely given orally despite its extensive first-pass metabolism and low bioavailability. Some results suggest that nasal absorption of the drug is by a process of passive diffusion[37]; however, extensive absorption of the dissociated species has led to adoption of the aqueous pores theory as an explanation.

It was suggested by Fisher and coworkers[10] that the aqueous pores within the nasal mucosa are considerably larger than those associated with the jejunum, which are believed to be of the order of 0.4–0.8 nm[38]. They observed that molecules as large as inulin and dextran (mol.wt 70 000) were excreted in bile and urine following their application to the nasal mucosa of anaesthetized rats. Inulin was significantly absorbed over a period of 6 h and dextran (although absorption was less dramatic) was detectable in bile and urine for that entire period.

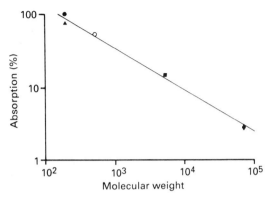

Figure 1.12 Correlation between percentage dose absorbed after nasal administration and molecular weight: 4-oxo-4*H*-1-benzopyran-2-carboxylic acid (●); *p*-aminohippuric acid (▲); sodium cromoglycate (○); inulin (■), and dextran (♦); $r = -0.996$. (From reference 39)

Fisher *et al.* [39] provided evidence to support the concept of diffusion via aqueous pores and suggested that such pores appear to be sufficiently large to facilitate the diffusion of inulin and dextrans (Figure 1.12).

Labile drugs

The acidic environment of the stomach tends rapidly to degrade many labile drugs, e.g. benzyl penicillin and peptides; the latter are, in addition, subject to enzymatic degradation by epithelial aminopeptidases. Consequently, alternative routes of administration have been sought for these drugs.

In recent years, peptides have become increasingly important as therapeutic agents and this has been paralleled by development of extremely potent hormone analogues. Because of the labile nature of these drugs, nasal administration appears to be a feasible alternative to the parenteral route and, indeed, has been investigated for vasopressin [40], growth hormone analogues [41] and other analogues of TRH [42] and LHRH [5]. Development of potential nasal formulations is often hindered by the very low absorption of these compounds, although this problem may be partly circumvented by synthesis of highly potent peptide analogues.

LHRH, a decapeptide, and its analogues have been used in the treatment of various endocrine disorders including hypogonadism and amenorrhoea [43]. It has been shown that 2 mg intranasal LH/FSHRH provides plasma levels that are equivalent to 100 μg delivered intravenously [43], a bioavailability of some 5%. Better nasal bioavailability has been reported by Sandow and Petri [42], who demonstrated that up to 20% of nasally administered TRH could be absorbed; however, these bioavailability values are the exception rather than the rule.

Nafarelin is a 'super-agonist' of LHRH, which displays >200 times the potency of the native peptide, and has been administered nasally to monkeys as a means of oestrus suppression: 250 μg nafarelin per day was sufficient to prevent pre-ovulatory surges of LH and oestrogen, to reduce progesterone to baseline levels and to prevent ovulation [12], an effect equivalent to 5 μg daily by i.m. injection (Figure 1.13). In similar types of experiments the effectiveness of nasal buserelin, a nanopeptide with 70 times the potency of LHRH, was investigated in women [44,45]. In all but two cases, 400 μg daily inhibited ovulation. In a subjective assessment the women reported that the nasal spray was convenient and practical, and the treatment free from side-effects.

Nasal administration of larger peptides has also been reported. Adrenocorticotrophic hormone (ACTH) contains 39

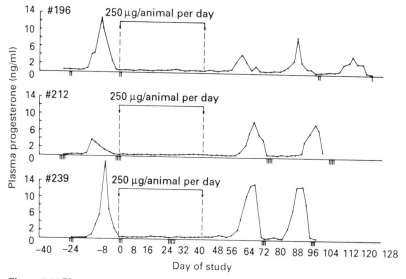

Figure 1.13 Plasma progesterone levels and menstrual flow patterns in three female rhesus monkeys before, during and after 42 days of consecutive daily intranasal administration of 250 μg nafarelin. (From reference 12)

amino acids and has a molecular weight of about 4500. Significant blood levels were observed following nasal delivery of 10 mg and 20 mg, reaching a maximum after 4 h [46]. This was accompanied by transient, mild irritation of the nasal mucosa. In a similar experiment it was reported that absorption of the ACTH agonist, α^{1-18}-ACTH, was similar following intranasal, i.m. and subcutaneous (s.c.) administration [47].

The largest market in nasal delivery of polypeptides would be for an effective formulation of insulin. The molecule consists of two peptide chains (21 and 30 amino acids) and has a molecular weight of c. 6000. It is extensively hydrolysed in the stomach, as would be expected, but its potential for nasal delivery is further compromised by the fact that it undergoes proteolytic degradation during its absorption across the nasal mucosa [48]. Consequently, nasal administration of insulin currently focuses on the use of penetration enhancers to promote uptake. This problem is discussed further later in this chapter (page 20).

Nasal drug delivery systems

It was suggested by Proctor [49] that 'water-soluble drugs are preferable for nasal delivery as the probability of achieving effective absorption from non-water-soluble drugs is limited'. However, as previously discussed, this generalization is invalid because several very lipophilic drugs (e.g. buprenorphine) are rapidly and extensively absorbed following nasal administration. Similarly, many ionized drug molecules are nasally absorbed (e.g. benzoic acid). Each drug being considered for nasal administration must therefore be taken on its merits, without any assumptions being made.

It was noted by Aoki and Crawley [18] that nasal distribution of radiolabelled albumin was markedly better following dosing of drops to supine subjects than spray-dosing to seated subjects. This was confirmed by Hardy et al. [17] who observed that administration of multiple small volumes was more effective than a single large volume (Figure 1.7). However as it is impractical for patients to prostrate themselves at regular and frequent intervals throughout the day, mechanical pump and aerosol systems are widely used in practice despite their poorer nasal distribution; for instance Beconase Aqueous and Beconase (Allen and Hanburys) are, respectively, spray and aerosol systems that deliver 50 µg beclomethasone dipropionate per actuation.

Both spray and aerosol systems are generally presented as sealed units, and in formulating such nasal delivery devices a number of points must be considered:

1. The drug (and enhancer if present) must be uniformly dispersed within the container;
2. If the drug is soluble in the propellant system, potential problems such as oxidation and the influence of pH fluctuations will be largely avoided. In some instances, however, separation of propellant and cosolvent may occur, in which case dose uniformity will not be maintained. Water-soluble drugs have been successfully formulated as solution, suspension and emulsion systems [50];
3. As discussed previously, the particle size distribution of aerosols can have a profound effect on intranasal distribution, and therefore on absorption. A diameter of at least 10 µm is required to ensure that loss into the lungs is minimized [1]. In addition, the velocity of ejection of the dosage form must be carefully monitored.

Microspheres

Materials administered to ciliated regions of the nasal mucosa will tend to be cleared rapidly. However, if particulates can be directed to the non-ciliated anterior regions their residence time may be increased to >1 h [17]. Thus, it has been postulated that bioadhesive particles could be of potential advantage, especially for poorly absorbed drugs. Distribution, within the nasal sac, of three microsphere systems was compared with conventional powders and solutions by means of gamma scintigraphy [19]. Solution and powder were both cleared rapidly ($t_{1/2}$ 15 min) but the three microsphere systems displayed much greater residence times within the nasal cavity and had $t_{1/2}$ values of >3 h (Figure 1.14). The nasal retention of these materials is a result of their capacity to imbibe water and become mucoadhesive. This approach of increasing contact time has been utilized by others: the absorption of nasally administered insulin in dogs was markedly enhanced by its formulation with gelling agents such as hydroxypropylcellulose and polyacrylic acid [51], and a polyacrylic acid gel for promotion of the absorption of insulin and calcitonin in rats has been described [52].

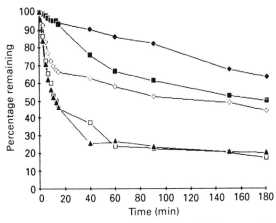

Figure 1.14 The clearance of three radio-labelled microsphere preparations (♦, DEAE-Sephadex; ■, starch; ◊, albumin) applied to volunteers by means of a nasal spray. Two control formulations (powder and solution, □, ▲) are included for comparison. (From reference 19)

Insulin

Currently, the only treatment available for Type 1 diabetic patients is daily administration of insulin by s.c. injection. Unfortunately, local discomfort, irritation and inconvenience make compliance a problem in some patients. Recently, efforts have been focused on the search for an enhancer that will promote nasal absorption to significant levels: compounds examined have included non-ionic surfactants[13] and bile salts[15]. Although bile salts have been shown to be reasonably successful[22], both these potential enhancers are toxic to mucous membranes[13, 53], and their daily administration would probably be associated with extreme irritation and toxicity. Despite these potential problems, mixed solutions of insulin and bile salts have been administered to humans in the form of a nasal spray containing 1% deoxycholate[54]. Serum levels peaked at 10 min and this was accompanied by a 50% reduction in blood glucose levels; bioavailability was estimated at 1–20% of an intravenous dose (Figure 1.15).

The most promising adjuvant for nasal delivery of insulin currently appears to be sodium taurodihydrofusidate (STDHF), a derivative of sodium fusidate. It has been suggested that expanded micelles of insulin–STDHF are produced, supplying a large reservoir of soluble insulin monomers that serve to

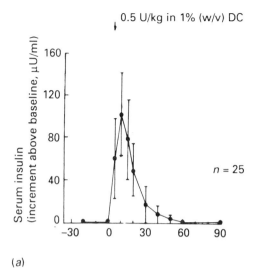

(a)

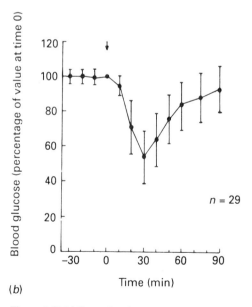

(b)

Figure 1.15 (a) Serum levels of insulin in normal volunteers after 0.5 U/kg of insulin in 1% w/v deoxycholate (DC) (mean ± SD; $n = 25$). (b) Changes in blood glucose level as a percentage of initial values following administration of 0.5 U/kg insulin in 1% w/v DC (mean ± SD; $n = 29$). (From reference 54)

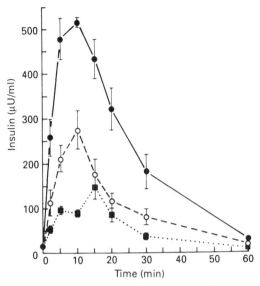

Figure 1.16 Kinetics of insulin absorption following nasal dosing with
(· · · ■ · · ·) 0.25, (– – ○ – –) 0.5 and (—●—) 1.0 U/kg, each preparation
containing 1% w/v sodium taurodihydrofusidate. (From reference 4)

promote absorption. Intranasal administration of the insulin–STDHF complex (containing 1% STDHF and varying doses of insulin) gave rise to rapid serum levels of insulin, with peak levels developing in only 10 min [4]. This type of profile mimics the kinetic pattern of endogenous insulin, where secretion tends to be pulsatile in response to ingested food, etc. (Figure 1.16). On the other hand, subcutaneous insulin produces a delayed onset of action, with greater variability in serum levels, and cannot reproduce the postprandial pulsing pattern. STDHF appears to be well tolerated by the nasal mucosa; it is apparently non-mutagenic and displays low levels of haemolytic potential.

Implications of nasal drug delivery

It is unlikely that nasal delivery will ever replace the oral route as the route of choice. However, there are many instances in which the oral route is contraindicated, e.g. for extensively metabolized drugs or acid-labile drugs. The nasal route has been shown to be viable for administration of metabolized drugs, e.g. naloxone[33], and labile drugs, e.g. enkephalins[11], and when a rapid onset of action is required, e.g. insulin[4]. However, there are many potential problems associated with formulating a drug for the nasal route. The ciliated nasal epithelial cells are part of the body's defences, in that inspired air is trapped in the turbinates and contaminants are removed via the cilia[49]. Although infrequent dosing of drugs is not likely to damage the epithelium and cilia extensively, chronic applications may lead to problems of irritancy and toxicity, and may ultimately damage the cilia and compromise the body's defences[55].

Nasal formulations are presented almost exclusively as multidose preparations, and therefore preservatives are required to prevent microbial contamination. Mercurial compounds appear to be most toxic (e.g. thiomersal), followed by lipophilic molecules such as chlorbutol. Polar preservatives possess the best characteristics, and a system containing 0.01% benzalkonium chloride and 0.05% EDTA has been recommended[55]. Local toxicity to the nasal mucosa must not be overlooked, because even transient damage may lead to infection. It follows that all formulation adjuvants must be shown to be safe before they are approved for chronic nasal administration, and routine histological examination of treated nasal mucosae should be undertaken. This also applies to penetration enhancers, the usefulness of which depends on exerting some local effect; some enhancers can induce extensive epithelial lysis, e.g. cholic acid[53].

The delivery of reproducible and accurate doses of drug solution can also be problematical. Hardy et al.[17] dosed human volunteers with 100 µl from a nasal spray and observed that at least ten actuations were required to provide good reproducibility of volume, and >20 were required to provide the full 100 µl. This inaccuracy of dispensed volume has been a great problem, and is of particular concern when highly potent drugs (e.g. peptides) are being administered. Currently, extensive research into the design of metered-dose nebulizers is being undertaken by pharmaceutical manufacturers. In one instance a system based on compressed nitrogen was originally devised. However, this was prone to leaks and was inaccurate (50% error was usual) and was therefore replaced by a spray system, in which inaccuracies of volume became apparent only when the container was tilted. Eventually a nebulizer was developed to provide reproducible and accurate dosing of peptides, even when tilted during actuation[56]. The improved nebulizer was extensively tested for the following features, which should be applied to any metered-dose, nebulized formulation: uniformity of droplet size and volume; accuracy of metered volume; batch-to-batch accuracy of metered volume; no adsorption of drug on to pump components; physical stability of formulation; sterility, and protection against bacterial contamination.

Because of poor aqueous solubility, or stability problems, some drugs cannot be formulated as aqueous sprays. The alternative systems, pressurized aerosols, tend to be complex, often containing several components in addition to the drug, e.g. water, cosolvent, preservatives and propellants. Thus, even before consideration of the design of the aerosol container, it is important to establish the physical stability of the formulation, including such parameters as crystal growth and polymorphism, and phase separation[7]. Propellants must be chosen carefully. In addition to physical stability considerations (propellants may act as solvents), the propellants must be expelled at an accurate and reproducible volume, even when the container is almost empty. Thus, vapour pressure of the propellant combination is an important formulation criterion. With the recent upsurge of public interest in environmental issues, it is likely that pharmaceutical formulators will come under increasing pressure to develop and use non-chlorofluorocarbon propellant systems.

The nasal route may be chosen for a particular drug because of its degradation in the GI tract. Many peptide and protein species (e.g. somatostatin and interleukins) are faced with an enzymatic barrier to absorption, and this is obviously an important contributor to their low bioavailability[57]. A study was undertaken by Stratford and Lee[58] in which they compared the aminopeptidase activities of epithelial cell supernatants extracted from various mucosal regions of the rabbit (Figure 1.17). It was apparent that the aminopeptidase activity in nasal mucosa was very similar to that in the duodenum, although not as intense as in the ileum, suggesting that nasally administered peptides are as prone to degradation as those administered orally. However, it must be remembered that these results were not obtained from intact functional epithelia, and that the degradative influences of gastric acid and proteolytic enzymes were not considered. Results of this nature from studies *in vitro* should not be considered in isolation because, irrespective of what such results appear to indicate, nasally administered peptides and proteins are often highly efficacious[4, 5, 15, 22, 59].

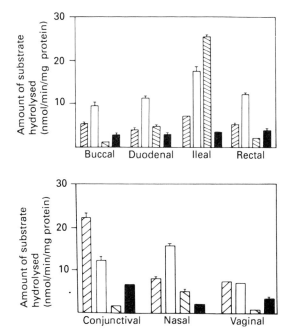

Figure 1.17 Mucosal aminopeptidase activity (in nmol substrate hydrolysed per min per mg protein) in the albino rabbit against four L-amino acid-4-methoxy-2-naphthylamide substrates. Substrates (1 mM concentration) were: L-leucine (▨), L-alanine (☐), L-glutamic acid (▥) and L-arginine (■). (From reference 58)

Conclusions

Nasal drug delivery is not an easy option, and is never likely to replace the oral route for routine administration. Probably the main potential problems relate to the small surface area of the nasal mucosa and the short residence times available for dosage forms. Consequently, only potent drugs, in non-irritant and non-toxic dosage forms, are likely to be candidates for this route of administration.

Few problems appear to be associated with use of the nasal route for treatment of local disorders such as allergic rhinitis and nasal congestion. Modern methods of chemical synthesis now provide many biologically active peptides, proteins and other labile molecules for which systemic administration via the nasal mucosa offers a potential means of bypassing acidic and enzymatic degradation in the GI tract. Many results have not been encouraging [5, 11, 12], and clearly a great deal of further work is required in order that poorly absorbed drugs may ultimately be delivered by this route. The use of penetration enhancers [4, 13] and mucoadhesive dosage forms [19] continue to be examined as means of improving absorption, but drug instability, dose uniformity and vehicle toxicity also continue to be problems that are difficult to overcome.

From the point of view of the patient, the nasal route is clearly preferable to parenteral administration, and the aim of many research groups is the development of an acceptable nasal formulation for insulin, calcitonin and other similarly labile drugs. There is little doubt that suitable formulations for systemic drug delivery via the nasal route will become available in the near future, patient acceptability and preference providing some of the impetus for the research and development required.

References

1. Proctor, D. F. The upper airways. I. Nasal physiology and defense of the lung. *American Review of Respiratory Disease*, 115, 97–129, 1977
2. Brain, J. D. and Valberg, P. A. Deposition of aerosol in the respiratory tract. *American Review of Respiratory Disease*, 120, 1325–1337, 1979
3. Skoogh, B. E., Simonsson, B. G., Berggren, A. G., Bergström, Z. and Johansson, M. Climate and environmental change in patients with chronic airway obstruction. *Archives of Environmental Health*, 31, 15–18, 1976
4. Longenecker, J. P. Nazlin® – transnasal systemic delivery of insulin. In *Delivery Systems for Peptide Drugs* (eds. S. S. Davis, L. Illum and E. Tomlinson), Plenum Press, New York, pp. 211–220, 1986
5. Anik, S. T., McRae, G., Nevenberg, C., Worden, A., Foreman, J., Hway, J. Y., Kushinsky, S., Jones, R. E. and Vickery, B. Nasal absorption of nafarelin acetate, the decapeptide [D-Nal (2)⁶] LHRH, in rhesus monkey. *Journal of Pharmaceutical Sciences*, 73, 684–685, 1984
6. Hirai, S., Takatsuka, Y., Tai, M. and Hiroyuki, M. Absorption of drugs from the nasal mucosa of rats. *International Journal of Pharmaceutics*, 7, 317–325, 1981
7. Su, K. S. E. and Campanale, K. M. Nasal drug delivery systems – requirements, developments, evaluations. In *Transnasal Systemic Medications* (ed. Y. W. Chien), Elsevier, Amsterdam, pp. 221–232, 1985
8. Hussain, A. A., Bawarshi-Nassar, R. and Huang, C. H. Physicochemical considerations in intranasal drug administration. In *Transnasal Systemic Medications* (ed. Y. W. Chien), Elsevier, Amsterdam, pp. 121–138, 1985
9. Hussain, A. A., Hirai, S. and Bawarshi, R. Nasal absorption of propranolol in rats. *Journal of Pharmaceutical Sciences*, 68, 1196, 1979
10. Fisher, A. N., Brown, K., Davis, S. S., Parr, G. D. and Smith, D. A. The nasal absorption of sodium cromoglycate in the albino rat. *Journal of Pharmacy and Pharmacology*, 37, 38–41, 1985

11. Su, K. S. E., Campanale, K. M., Mendelsohn, L. G., Kerchner, G. A. and Gries, C. L. Nasal delivery of polypeptides. I: nasal absorption of enkephalins. *Journal of Pharmaceutical Sciences*, **74**, 394–398, 1985
12. Vickery, B., Anik, S. T., Chaplin, M. and Henzl, M. Intranasal administration of nafarelin acetate – contraception and therapeutic application. In *Transnasal Systemic Medications* (ed. Y. W. Chien), Elsevier, Amsterdam, pp. 210–216, 1985
13. Hirai, S., Yashiki, T. and Mima, H. Mechanisms for the enhancement of the nasal absorption of insulin by surfactants. *International Journal of Pharmaceutics*, **9**, 317–325, 1981
14. Hussain, A. A., Hirai, S. and Bawarshi, R. Nasal absorption of propranolol from different dosage forms by rats and dogs. *Journal of Pharmaceutical Sciences*, **69**, 1411–1413, 1980
15. Moses, A. C., Gordon, G. S., Carey, M. C. and Flier, J. S. Insulin administered intranasally as an insulin–bile salt aerosol: effectiveness and reproducibility in normal and diabetic subjects. *Diabetes*, **32**, 1040–1047, 1983
16. Johnson, P. E., Greenberg, S. B., Harmon, M. W., Alford, B. R. and Couch, R. B. Recovery of applied human leukocyte interferon from the nasal mucosa of chimpanzees and humans. *Journal of Clinical Microbiology*, **4**, 106–110, 1976
17. Hardy, J. G., Lee, S. W. and Wilson, C. G. Intranasal drug delivery by sprays and drops. *Journal of Pharmacy and Pharmacology*, **37**, 294–297, 1985
18. Aoki, Y. F. and Crawley, J. C. W. Distribution and removal of human serum albumin–technetium 99m administered intranasally. *British Journal of Clinical Pharmacology*, **3**, 869–878, 1976
19. Illum, L. Microspheres as a potential controlled release nasal drug delivery system. In *Delivery Systems for Peptide Drugs* (eds S. S. Davis, L. Illum and E. Tomlinson), Plenum Press, New York, pp. 205–210, 1986
20. Rigg, L. A., Milanes, B., Villanueva, B. and Yen, S. S. C. Efficacy of intravaginal and intranasal administration of micronised estradiol-17β. *Journal of Clinical Endocrinology and Metabolism*, **45**, 1261–1264, 1977
21. Hoover, R. T. Intranasal oxytocin in eighteen-hundred patients. *American Journal of Obstetrics and Gynecology*, **110**, 788–794, 1971
22. Pontiroli, A. E., Alberetto, M., Secchi, A., Dossi, G., Bosi, I. and Pozza, G. Insulin given intranasally induces hypoglycaemia in normal and diabetic subjects. *British Medical Journal*, **284**, 303–306, 1982
23. Van Dyke, C., Jatlow, P., Ungerer, J., Barash, P. and Byck, R. Cocaine and lidocaine have similar psychological effects after intranasal application. *Life Sciences*, **24**, 271–274, 1979
24. Tonndorf, J., Chinn, H. I. and Lett, J. E. Absorption from nasal mucous membrane: systemic effect of hyoscine following intranasal administration. *Annals of Otology, Rhinology and Laryngology*, **62**, 630–634, 1953
25. Hendricks, C. and Gabel, R. A. Use of intranasal oxytocin in obstetrics. I. Laboratory evaluation. *American Journal of Obstetrics and Gynecology*, **79**, 780–788, 1960
26. Hill, A. B., Bowley, C. J., Nahrwold, M. L., Knight, P. R., Kirsh, M. M. and Denlinger, J. K. Intranasal administration of nitroglycerin. *Anesthesiology*, **51**, S 67, 1979
27. Chien, Y. W. and Chang, S. F. Historic development of transnasal systemic medication. In *Transnasal Systemic Medication* (ed. Y. W. Chien), Elsevier, Amsterdam, pp. 1–99, 1985
28. Cho, M. J., Thompson, D. P., Cramer, C. T., Vidmar, T. J. and Scieszka, J. F. The Madin Darby canine kidney (MDCK) epithelial cell monolayer as a model cellular transport barrier. *Pharmaceutical Research*, **6**, 71–77, 1989

29. Shand, D. G., Nuckolls, E. M. and Oates, J. A. Plasma propranolol levels in adults with observations in four children. *Clinical Pharmacology and Therapeutics*, **11**, 112–120, 1970
30. Hussain, A. A., Foster, T., Hirai, S., Kashihara, T., Batenhorst, R. and Jones, M. Nasal absorption of propranolol in humans. *Journal of Pharmaceutical Sciences*, **69**, 1240, 1980
31. Van de Donk, H. J. M. and Merkus, F. W. H. M. Decrease in ciliary beat frequency due to intranasal administration of propranolol. *Journal of Pharmaceutical Sciences*, **71**, 595–596, 1982
32. Brewster, D., Humphrey, M. J. and McLeavy, M. A. The systemic bioavailability of buprenorphine by various routes of administration. *Journal of Pharmacy and Pharmacology*, **33**, 500–506, 1981
33. Hussain, A. A., Kimura, R., Huang, C. M. and Kashihara, T. Nasal absorption of naloxone and buprenorphine in rats. *International Journal of Pharmaceutics*, **21**, 233–237, 1984
34. Anand Kumar, T. C., David, G. F. X., Uberkoman, B. and Saini, K. D. Uptake of radioactivity by body fluid and tissues in rhesus monkeys after intravenous injection or intranasal spray of tritium-labelled oestradiol and progesterone. *Current Science*, **43**, 435–439, 1974
35. Anand Kumar, T. C., David, G. F. X. and Puri, V. Nasal sprays for controlling ovulation in rhesus monkey. In *Recent Advances in Primatology, Vol. 4* (eds. D. J. Chivers and E. H. R. Ford), Academic Press, London, pp. 142–160, 1978
36. Ho, N. F. H., Higuchi, W. I. and Turi, J. Theoretical model studies of drug absorption and transport in the G.I. tract. *Journal of Pharmaceutical Sciences*, **61**, 192–197, 1972
37. Kaneo, Y. Absorption from the rat mucous membrane. I. Nasal absorption of hydrallazine in rats. *Acta Pharmaceutica Suecica*, **20**, 379–383, 1983
38. Hyashi, M., Hirasawa, T., Muraska, T., Shiga, M. and Awazu, S. Comparison of water influx and sieving coefficient in rat jejunal, nasal and rectal absorptions of antipyrene. *Chemical and Pharmaceutical Bulletin*, **33**, 2149–2152, 1985
39. Fisher, A. N., Brown, K., Davis, S. S., Parr, G. D. and Smith, D. A. The effect of molecular size on the nasal absorption of water-soluble compounds in the albino rat. *Journal of Pharmacy and Pharmacology*, **39**, 357–362, 1987
40. Cobb, W. E., Spare, S. and Reichlin, S. Neurogenic diabetes insipidus: management with DDAVP (1-desamino-8-D-arginine vasopressin). *Annals of Internal Medicine*, **88**, 183–188, 1978
41. Evans, W. S., Borges, J. L. C., Kaiser, D. L., Vance, M. L., Sellers, R. P., MacLeod, R. M., Vale, W., Rivier, J. and Thorner, M. O. Intranasal administration of human pancreatic tumor GH-releasing factor-40 stimulates GH release in normal men. *Journal of Clinical Endocrinology and Metabolism*, **57**, 1081–1083, 1983
42. Sandow, J. and Petri, W. Intranasal administration of peptides – biological activity and therapeutic efficacy. In *Transnasal Systemic Medication* (ed. Y. W. Chien), Elsevier, Amsterdam, pp. 183–200, 1985
43. Zatuchni, G. I., Shelton, J. D. and Sciarra, J. J. (eds). *LHRH Peptides as Female and Male Contraceptives*, Harper and Row, Philadelphia, 1976
44. Jeppsson, S., Kullander, S., Rannevik, G. and Thorelli, J. Intranasal administration of synthetic gonadotrophin-releasing hormone. *British Medical Journal*, **4**, 231, 1973
45. Bergquist, C., Nillies, S. J. and Wide, L. Intranasal gonadotrophin-releasing hormone agonist as a contraceptive agent. *Lancet*, **ii**, 215–216, 1979

46. Smith, R. W., Dickson, L. C., Bryan, J. B. and Lowrie, W. D. Nasal administration of ACTH: observations of effectiveness measured by blood eosinopenic response. *Journal of Clinical Endocrinology and Metabolism*, **12**, 958–959, 1952

47. Keenan, J., Thompson, J. B., Chamberlain, M. A. and Besser, G. M. Prolonged corticotrophic action of a synthetic substituted α^{1-18}ACTH. *British Medical Journal*, **3**, 742–743, 1971

48. Smith, E. L., Hill, R. L. and Borman, A. Activity of insulin degraded by leucine aminopeptidases. *Biochimica et biophysica acta*, **29**, 207–208, 1958

49. Proctor, D. G. Nasal physiology in intranasal drug administrations. In *Transnasal Systemic Medications* (ed. Y. W. Chien), Elsevier, Amsterdam, pp. 100–106, 1985

50. Sciarra, J. J. and Stoller, L. *The Science and Technology of Aerosol Packaging*, Wiley, New York, pp. 429–450, 1974

51. Nagai, T., Nishimoto, Y., Nambu, N., Suzuki, Y. and Sekine, K. Powder dosage form of insulin for nasal administration. *Journal of Controlled Release*, **1**, 15–22, 1984

52. Morimoto, K., Morisaka, K. and Kamada, A. Enhancement of nasal absorption of insulin and calcitonin using polyacrylic acid gel. *Journal of Pharmacy and Pharmacology*, **37**, 134–136, 1985

53. Martin, G. P. and Marriott, C. Membrane damage by bile salts: the protective function of phospholipids. *Journal of Pharmacy and Pharmacology*, **33**, 754–759, 1981

54. Flier, J. S., Moses, A. C., Carey, M. C., Gordon, G. S. and Silver, R. S. Intranasal administration of insulin – efficacy and mechanisms. In *Transnasal Systemic Medications* (ed. Y. W. Chien), Elsevier, Amsterdam, pp. 217–226, 1985

55. Hermens, W. A. J. J. and Merkus, F. W. H. M. The influence of drugs on nasal ciliary movement. *Pharmaceutical Research*, **4**, 445–449, 1987

56. Petri, W., Schmiedel, R. and Sandow, J. Development of a metered-dose nebuliser for intranasal peptide administration. In *Transnasal Systemic Medications* (ed. Y. W. Chien), Elsevier, Amsterdam, pp. 161–182, 1985

57. Okada, H., Yamazaki, I., Ogawa, Y., Hirai, S., Yashiki, T. and Mima, H. J. Vaginal absorption of a potent LHRH analog (Leuprolide) in rats. I: absorption by various routes and absorption enhancement. *Journal of Pharmaceutical Sciences*, **71**, 1367–1371, 1982

58. Stratford, R. E. and Lee, V. H. L. Aminopeptidase activity in homogenates of various absorptive mucosae in the albino rabbit: implications in peptide delivery. *International Journal of Pharmaceutics*, **30**, 73–82, 1986

59. Lider, A. S., Holland, F. J., Costigan, D. C., Jenner, M. R., Wielgosz, G. and Fazekas, A. T. A. Intranasal and subcutaneous treatment of central, precocious puberty in both sexes with a long acting analog of luteinizing hormone-releasing hormone. *Journal of Clinical Endocrinology and Metabolism*, **58**, 966–969, 1984

Further reading

Chien, Y. W. (ed.) *Transnasal Systemic Medications*, Elsevier, Amsterdam, 1985

Davis, S. S., Illum, L. and Tomlinson, E. (eds) *Delivery Systems for Peptide Drugs*, Plenum Press, New York, 1986

2

Buccal and sublingual delivery of drugs

P.-J. Lamey and M. A. O. Lewis

Introduction

> *". . .il suffit d'en tenir une très-petite quantité*
> *sur la langue pour en éprouver une migraine*
> *assez forte pendant plusieurs heures."**

Ascagne Sobrero, 1847

The above extract is taken from the first paper to describe the systemic effects of a drug (nitroglycerin) applied topically to the mouth[1]. However, this early clinical observation was questioned by many and it was not until some 30 years later, following the introduction of nitroglycerin drops for the treatment of angina, that lingual administration became accepted. Since that time the usefulness of administering a number of other drugs has been investigated[2].

There are two principal sites within the oral cavity which may be used for drug absorption: these are the sublingual region, where a therapeutic agent is placed under the tongue, and the buccal region, where the medicine is held between the cheek (or lip) and the gingivae adjacent to the teeth. The potential advantages of drug delivery via the oral mucosa are avoidance of first-pass liver metabolism, elimination of exposure to gastrointestinal fluids and no delay in absorption attributable to the presence of food or gastric disease. In addition, drugs can be administered in this way to unconscious patients.

Although the oral cavity may appear to be an ideal site for drug administration, unfortunately not all drugs are able to penetrate the oral mucosa. Other disadvantages are that

*'. . . it's enough to have a very small quantity on the tongue to result in a very bad migraine which lasts several hours.'

maintenance of the dosage form at the sublingual or buccal sites is difficult, and clearly both are of smaller surface area than the duodenum. There is also variation between patients in their compliance and other factors such as salivary flow and rate of drug absorption.

Anatomy of the oral cavity

The oral mucosa

The oral cavity is lined by a permeable mucous membrane with an underlying connective tissue[3]. The corium has extensive venous and lymphatic drainage, factors which make the mouth a suitable site for the topical administration of drugs for systemic effect.

The oral mucosa, like skin, consists of stratified squamous epithelium but, unlike skin, it is described as a mucous membrane because it is lubricated and protected by saliva. Most of the lining, consisting of the cheeks, lips, soft palate, floor of mouth and ventral surface of tongue, is composed of a simple mucous membrane (Figure 2.1a). The hard palate, dorsal surface of tongue and tissues immediately adjacent to the teeth are exposed to the mechanical irritation of mastication and are thickened by a layer of keratin similar to that found in skin (Figure 2.1b). As the stratum corneum may be a potential barrier to mucosal penetration, drugs are traditionally placed at non-keratinized sites.

The surface area of the mouth available for drug absorption is approximately $200\,cm^2$; because of the small size of the oral cavity (compared with the gut) only potent drugs (usually in a small tablet form) are likely to be effective when administered in this way. Although emphasis has been placed on the structural differences between keratinized and non-keratinized oral mucosae, there is no compelling evidence for major differences between them in drug absorption capabilities. Studies using peroxidase and lanthanum have shown equivalent impermeability in keratinized and non-keratinized oral epithelia. The conclusion from these studies, and others using electrolytes, was that rather than the keratinized surface layer representing a barrier, it was the presence of membrane-coating granules that was important. In addition, intercellular junctions did not seem to influence permeability whereas the intercellular space itself, although only a minor (1%) component of tissue volume, could do so. The ingress of electrolytes and lipid-insoluble substances

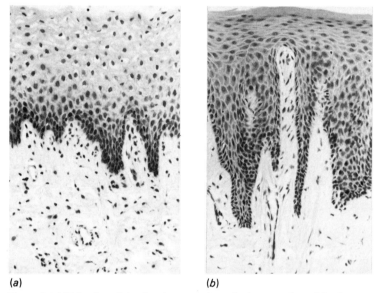

(a)   (b)

Figure 2.1 (a) Non-keratinized oral mucosa from the inner surface of the lip. (b) Keratinized oral mucosa from the hard palate. (Courtesy of Dr D. G. MacDonald, Glasgow Dental Hospital and School)

by this pathway suggests that superficial layers could be traversed.

In certain circumstances there may be differences in permeability between keratinized and non-keratinized oral epithelium, as increased permeability of non-keratinized oral epithelium to water has been reported. Other factors that may be important include mucosal disease or thinning of the oral epithelium. Certainly, the sublingual epithelium is slightly thinner than buccal epithelium, and its immersion in saliva would tend to give it an increased permeability to most substances.

Venous and lymphatic drainage

The tissues of the oral cavity are highly vascular and, as venous drainage from the mouth is to the superior vena cava (Figure 2.2), any absorbed drug is protected from rapid first-pass metabolism in the liver (Figure 2.3). The richness of the blood and lymphatic supply and drainage is a major factor in the rapidity of systemic drug effect following absorption. The oral cavity is also bathed in saliva (pH 6.2–7.4) and therefore

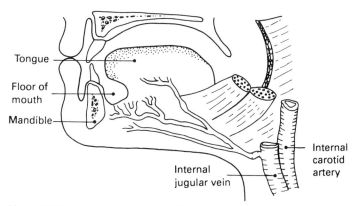

Figure 2.2 Venous drainage from the floor of the mouth

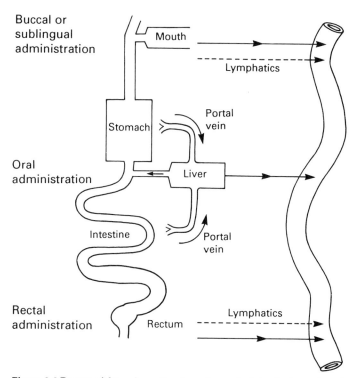

Figure 2.3 Routes of drug absorption from the gastrointestinal tract into the general circulation

relatively large amounts of 'water' are present. This overcomes one of the problems of rectal drug administration, where the small amount of fluid available for drug dissolution is a critical factor in absorption. Although the venous system and capillaries are probably of greater significance for systemic absorption, in some circumstances (such as the buccal administration of *para*-aminosalicylic acid in rabbits) uptake into lymphatics also occurs.

Physiology of drug absorption from the oral cavity

Some general comments can be made in relation to sublingual and buccal drug absorption. First, this route has not been studied to the same extent as other routes of drug administration[4]. Secondly, drugs have generally been studied in tablet form, although solutions, aerosols and pastes have also received some attention. Thirdly, it is important that during drug administration the patient does not indulge in activities (e.g. talking, drinking, smoking, etc.) that might affect 'residence time', the period that the drug is in direct contact with the mucosa. In addition, because salivary 'flow rate' is important in determining the rate of dissolution of the drug, it is important that the latter has a bland taste in order not to promote saliva flow; excessive saliva production will increase the likelihood of part of the drug being swallowed before absorption. Residence time is important and may be directly related to the formulation of the drug; solutions will have a shorter residence time than tablets, and patients should be encouraged to allow the latter to dissolve without sucking them.

Lipid solubility of the drug is important in that moderately lipophilic drugs are well absorbed, but if the drug is too water-insoluble, absorption is restricted. Solutions of drugs are generally better absorbed than suspensions because the first step in the process of absorption (namely dissolution, which may be rate-limiting) is obviated. Mention has already been made of salivary pH, which, having a value of *c*. 7, is important for both acidic and basic drug absorption. Another factor which must be considered is drug retention on cell membranes and the protein content of saliva, as both can interfere with absorption, particularly of drugs such as propranolol[5, 6].

A fundamental function of the oral mucosa is to produce an effective barrier to most potentially harmful substances. This property is achieved by the presence of an intact stratified squamous epithelium, similar to that in skin. However, unlike skin, the oral mucosa has a moist surface due to the presence of saliva. Although saliva assists the protective function against disease, it also increases the permeability of the mucosa as a result of surface hydration. However, the oral mucous membrane resembles skin more closely than gut in permeability and has a distinct advantage over parenteral and percutaneous routes for systemic delivery.

The physicochemical mechanisms involved in the transfer of drugs across the oral mucous membrane are similar to those at other cell membranes[4, 7]. Important factors related to the drug are molecular size and shape, solubility at the site of absorption, degree of ionization and lipid solubility. Drugs can cross the mucous membrane either by passive processes or by active processes.

Simple diffusion

Diffusion through a lipid phase is the major method by which substances transfer across the oral mucosa. The absorption pathway is based on the random motion of molecules from a zone of high concentration to one of low concentration. At first there is rapid passage but this gradually diminishes and rate of penetration is directly proportional to the concentration of the substance placed on the mucosa.

Intercellular movement

Depending on the nature of cell–cell junctions, epithelia have been described as either 'tight' or 'leaky'. The oral epithelium has a low population of tight junctions and could be regarded as leaky, and therefore is likely to allow passage of substances through intercellular spaces. The basal lamina is probably the limiting factor and restricts passage of molecules with a molecular weight >70 000 [7].

Endocytosis

The absorption of solid particles (phagocytosis) or of fluids (pinocytosis) are referred to collectively as endocytosis. Although cells of the oral mucosa are able to absorb substances by endocytosis it is likely that this mechanism has only a minor role in drug transport from the oral cavity.

Active transport

Metabolic energy is required to transport molecules or ions against a concentration or electrochemical gradient. Although it has been shown that this mechanism is involved in intestinal transport, it is unlikely that it is involved in the mouth.

The physical and chemical properties of a drug are the most important factors that determine its ability to penetrate the oral mucosa. Although there are exceptions, it is generally accepted that unionized molecules are absorbed more readily than ionic forms, and small molecules are more effectively absorbed than larger ones. The ability of the substance to dissolve in either non-polar (lipid) or polar (aqueous) solvents is also a major factor; although solubility in lipid is slightly more important, the ability to dissolve in both media leads to maximal passage. Degree of ionization of the drug is dependent on the environmental pH; passage of ionized substances, therefore, will be affected by the pH of saliva, as this will determine the degree of ionization.

Drugs given buccally or sublingually

It is now well recognized that therapeutic levels of certain drugs can be achieved in the systemic circulation if they are placed in contact with the oral mucosa. A major advantage of absorption by the oral mucosa is initial avoidance of the portal circulation and therefore possible inactivation of drug by first passage through the liver (first-pass effect). The application of a number of drugs in either tablet, lozenge, ointment or spray form has been investigated[2]; some drugs and formulations that are currently administered sublingually or buccally are listed in Table 2.1.

Cardioactive drugs

Glyceryl trinitrate and isosorbide dinitrate

Both these drugs are used for the treatment of angina pectoris, variant angina, congestive heart failure, acute myocardial infarction and peripheral vascular diseases[8]. They act by reducing venous return and thereby limit left ventricular work. They also cause vasodilatation of the coronary arteries. As well as having the advantage of rapidity of action, the buccal or sublingual delivery of these drugs can also be easily terminated.

Table 2.1 Examples of drugs and formulations administered buccally or sublingually in clinical practice

Drug	Formulation		Administration site
Buprenorphine hydrochloride	Tablet	: 200 µg	Sublingual
Ergotamine tartrate	Tablet	: 2 mg	Sublingual
Glyceryl trinitrate	Tablet	: 300–600 µg	Sublingual
	Aerosol spray	: 400 µg/metered dose	On or under tongue
	Sustained-release tablet	: 1–5 mg	Between upper labial mucosa and gingiva
Isosorbide dinitrate	Tablet	: 5–40 mg	Sublingual
	Chewable tablet	: 5 mg	Buccal
Nifedipine	Capsules	: 5–10 mg	Buccal (encapsulated liquid retained in mouth)
Phenazocine hydrobromide	Tablet	: 5 mg	Sublingual
Prochlorperazine maleate	Tablet	: 3 mg	Between upper labial mucosa and gingiva

Glyceryl trinitrate is non-ionic and has a very high lipid solubility. As the drug is very potent, relatively few molecules need to be absorbed to produce a therapeutic effect; the rich venous drainage of the mouth floor results in rapid transfer of the drug to the systemic circulation. Oral absorption of glyceryl trinitrate followed by passage through the liver produces a marked reduction in active drug in the circulation.

High serum levels of glyceryl trinitrate (Figure 2.4) and of isosorbide are achieved within 10 min of sublingual administration. However, the rate of elimination of both drugs is also rapid, so this route of therapy is suitable only for acute treatment. Maintenance and prophylactic therapy is achieved using oral administration; however, relatively high doses are required to overcome presystemic elimination [10].

Although glyceryl trinitrate was originally used in tablet form (Figure 2.5), other dosage forms [9, 10] including an aerosol spray preparation are now available [11] and provide an alternative method of treatment for those patients who find difficulty in holding sublingual preparations in position.

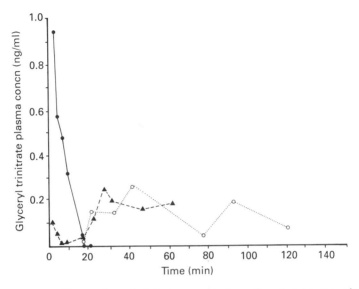

Figure 2.4 Plasma glyceryl trinitrate concentrations after administration of a 0.3 mg sublingual tablet (●), a 6.5 mg sustained-release oral capsule (○) and application of 16 mg as an ointment (▲). (Adapted from reference 9)

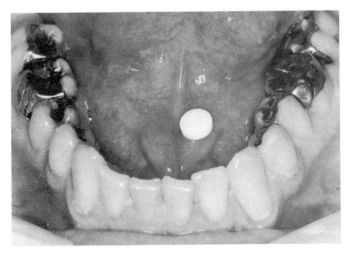

Figure 2.5 Glyceryl trinitrate tablet (300 µg) placed in the sublingual region

Nifedipine

Nifedipine is a calcium-channel blocker that interferes with the inward displacement of calcium ions through the slow channels of active cell membranes. This property is used to treat certain types of angina and hypertension by relaxing vascular smooth muscle, thereby dilating coronary and peripheral arteries. Peak concentrations of nifedipine are reached within 1 h of sublingual administration; therapeutic effects are rapid in onset and persist for c. 3 h following a 10 mg tablet[12]. However, it appears that the major site of nifedipine absorption is the stomach, and the advantages of sublingual administration are disputed[13, 14].

Propranolol

The absorption of this drug from the oral cavity has not been studied in detail but it is a good example of pH-dependent absorption[5]. It has been demonstrated with propranolol that 'buccal absorption' is not synonymous with 'systemic absorption' because back-partitioning (perhaps from stores in the thicker parts of the buccal membrane, cf. the sublingual membrane which is only a few cells thick) into saliva in the mouth can occur. After retaining a 200 µg dose in solution (pH 9.5) in the mouth for a few minutes, rinsing for 2 min with solutions of pH 9.0 and 5.2 resulted in recovery of about 19% and 55% of the 'absorbed' dose respectively[6].

Verapamil

Because this drug undergoes extensive first-pass metabolism, only 10–20% of an oral dose reaches the systemic circulation. Attempts have therefore been made to compare buccal absorption with oral and intravenous administration[15]. Although buccal administration was more efficacious than oral administration, bioavailability by both routes was equivalent (37% and 33% respectively). Such studies have led to the conclusion that other factors, such as storage and metabolism in the oral mucosa, greatly decrease the usefulness of buccal delivery.

Narcotic analgesics

Morphine

Morphine administered buccally is 40–50% more bioavailable than after intramuscular injection, and the adverse effects are milder[16].

Buprenorphine

Buprenorphine hydrochloride is a long-acting synthetic opioid analgesic which may be administered sublingually to relieve moderate to severe pain of various types, including osteoarthrosis, back pain, general injury, neurological pain, musculoskeletal pain and carcinoma. It should be prescribed with caution, however, because administration can cause dependence and tolerance, especially in patients with a history of narcotic dependence.

Sublingual administration is particularly useful as there is a substantial first-pass effect in the liver when buprenorphine is given orally. The approximate potency ratio of sublingual to oral is 1:10 and this relates to the high hepatic inactivation (85%) on first pass. Although the initial absorption is rapid, this subsequently diminishes and variations in peak plasma times can occur between individuals. Peak plasma concentrations following sublingual administration of 0.4 mg and 0.8 mg buprenorphine were achieved in a mean time of 200 min, with a range of 90–360 min (Figure 2.6). As absorption of buprenorphine is relatively slow from the sublingual site, administration of the drug by this route is suitable for maintenance of treatment

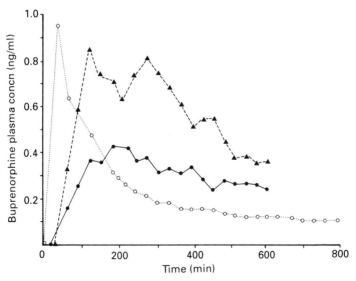

Figure 2.6 Mean plasma concentrations of buprenorphine after administration of 0.3 mg intravenously (O) and 0.4 mg (●) and 0.8 mg (▲) sublingually in two tablets. (Adapted from reference 17)

rather than for relief of acute episodes of pain; in acute situations, parenteral administration should be employed[18].

Phenazocine

Phenazocine hydrobromide is used sublingually to control severe pain[19]. It is particularly useful in the management of biliary colic as it has less tendency than other narcotic analgesics to increase biliary pressure. Sublingual administration is also useful if nausea and vomiting are a problem, or if upper gastrointestinal disease is present which may affect the absorption of drugs given orally. A 5 mg amount of phenazocine held in the buccal sulcus is as effective as 2 mg given intramuscularly in patients with postoperative pain. It has also been shown that sublingual administration is considerably more effective than oral doses. Large doses such as 10–20 mg applied sublingually twice daily are suitable for the control of pain associated with carcinoma.

Anti-migraine drugs

Ergotamine

The use of ergotamine is an accepted treatment for patients with migraine, especially those who do not respond to analgesics. The effectiveness of ergotamine in the treatment is based on its ability to constrict blood vessels. However, the use is limited due to side-effects of nausea, vomiting, abdominal pain and muscular cramps. It should not be used as prophylaxis for migraine nor should it be prescribed in doses >12 mg/week. Sublingual preparations are available for treatment of acute episodes, although it is not clear whether they are any more effective than tablets, suppositories or aerosol preparations[20]. The limited therapeutic use of buccal absorption of ergotamine is probably attributable to its low aqueous solubility at the pH of saliva[21].

Bronchodilators

Isoprenaline

Aerosol and sublingual tablet forms of isoprenaline salts are available for the treatment of reversible airway obstruction.

Neuroleptic drugs

Prochlorperazine

Prochlorperazine maleate is a piperazine derivative of pheno-thiazine used in the treatment of symptomatic vertigo due to Ménière's disease and labyrinthitis, nausea and vomiting from whatever cause, and in the management of migraine. Recently a buccal formulation of prochlorperazine has become available. Clinical assessment has shown that dosing three times daily with 3 mg by the buccal route is as effective as 5 mg by the oral route [22].

Experimental aspects of sublingual and buccal drug delivery

There have been several approaches to the study of this topic and these studies have involved both animals and man. The wide range of techniques and agents used makes comparison difficult but, in general, methods *in vivo* and *in vitro* have been employed [5, 7].

Studies *in vivo* have focused on local measurement of drug uptake or penetration through mucosal barriers. Frequently, these studies have been histological and involved the demonstration of altered capillary permeability, or alterations in epithelial mitotic activity, to topically applied agents. Such studies were limited by the necessity for biopsy; subsequent studies therefore used radioactive isotopes as a means of labelling the drug in the hope of providing greater sensitivity. Radio-labelling studies also offered the possibility of monitoring systemic uptake, in either blood or urine, and providing quantitative data.

Methods *in vitro* have the advantage of studying a defined anatomical region of oral mucosa. These techniques thus were considered an improvement on the buccal absorption test which, in fact, cannot provide information on the relative permeability of different areas of the oral mucosa as there is no means of determining the site of absorption.

The problem with experimentation *in vitro* has principally been one of technique. Parameters such as temperature can easily be controlled but considerable mechanical manipulation of tissue is required as these studies generally involve diffusion chambers. The data obtained from such studies are limited although they have provided basic information about factors influencing drug penetration through oral mucosa. For example, it has become clear that the physical and the chemical nature of the substance are the most important factors determining drug absorption[4, 5]. Ionic substances tend to pass less readily, as do large molecules. The pH of the surrounding media will also influence absorption depending on the pK_a of the drug. The concomitant administration of solvents or vehicles in which the drug is applied may also be important through alteration of surface hydration or intrinsic permeability of the surface mucosa.

Finally, comparisons between results *in vivo* and *in vitro* may require caution. Experimental studies on rabbits have suggested that substances of molecular weight *c.* 70 000 will cross non-keratinized oral mucosa *in vitro*, whereas substances of half this molecular weight do not penetrate *in vivo*.

Nalbuphine hydrochloride

This compound, a narcotic agonist/antagonist, is available in injectable form for relief of moderate to severe pain. Oral bioavailability is known to be low, because of the effect of first-pass metabolism in the gut and liver. However, animal experiments have shown that nalbuphine is rapidly absorbed after buccal administration and bioavailability is significantly improved. It is, therefore, possible that oral mucosal delivery may have an application in human patients.

Oestradiol

The absorption and effectiveness of sublingual administration of micronized 17-β-oestradiol (E_2) has been evaluated in the treatment of symptomatic postmenopausal women[23,24]. Although the sublingual route achieves peak serum levels of E_2 within an hour, there is also a rapid return to base levels. As E_2 levels drop there is an increase in the level of oestrone, presumably through conversion of E_2. However, as the sublingual route is more effective than the oral route, and because lower doses are involved, it may be preferable. Patients may also find a sublingual preparation preferable to topical vaginal creams. More work in this area seems to be indicated, but the development of orally effective oestrogenic drugs may limit this application.

Oxytocin

In the past there was a vogue for utilizing buccal oxytocin to induce and sustain labour. Several studies were reported and the popularity of this application increased, but criticism was made that it was of value only when the cervix was already ripe. In addition, it was considered too slow in onset, difficult to control and toxic effects were prolonged. These criticisms had some basis, as it was reported that the half-life was longer than after intravenous infusion, which has now replaced buccal delivery [25].

Heparin

Although early reports enthused about the benefits of sublingual delivery of heparin, the claims were soon retracted. Despite its large size, heparin is absorbed sublingually but the absorbed form has no effect on coagulation. Interestingly, heparin administered by this route does decrease postprandial serum lipids and this may have therapeutic implications.

Insulin

Research into the sublingual absorption of insulin has shown that, although it is not entirely inert when administered by this route, its efficacy is uncertain and therefore it cannot provide adequate glycaemic control.

Recently, a new mucosal dosage form of insulin was tested in dogs [26]. By combining the insulin with an adherent hydroxypropyl cellulose base, oral adhesion could be achieved for up to 6 h. The conclusions from these studies were that insulin could permeate the oral mucosa but only in the presence of sodium glycocholate. However, even in combination, the levels of insulin achieved compared poorly with those from parenteral or nasal administration.

Protirelin

Although much of the literature concerning sublingual and buccal drug absorption is not encouraging, there are claims that buccal protirelin is an effective means of stimulating thyrotropin and prolactin secretion [27]. One group of investigators concluded that buccal protirelin had many advantages over other methods of administration and advocated its use for diagnostic purposes.

Summary

The structure of the oral mucosa, coupled with the high degree of vascularity of the mouth, provides a readily accessible site for systemic administration of drugs. Sublingual or buccal delivery has the distinct advantage of avoiding exposure to gastric acids and passage through the liver. Although parenteral administration and rectal suppository formulations would overcome these problems, these routes are unacceptable to many patients. A number of factors, such as lipid solubility and ionization at the pH of saliva, influence the effectiveness of this route and few drugs are administered in this way. At present the main application of sublingual and buccal delivery is for rapid administration of potent drugs, for example glyceryl trinitrate, in the treatment of angina.

The vast majority of patients included in clinical trials of sublingual and buccal preparations have accepted these routes of administration without problems and patient compliance has been good. Although some patients have been aware of tasting products, this has been a minor complaint. There has been little work on development of optimal drug delivery systems for long-term sublingual or buccal use and further study seems indicated. Greater understanding of the permeability of the oral mucosa may result in the development of a larger number of drugs that can be administered to patients by these routes.

References

1. Sobrero, A. Sur plusieurs composés détonants produits avec l'acide nitrique et le sucre, la dextrine, la lactine, la mannite et la glycérine. *Comptes rendus hebdomadaires des séances de l'Académie des sciences*, **24**, 247–248, 1847
2. Editorial. Administration of drugs by the buccal route. *Lancet*, i, 666–667, 1987
3. Prime, S. Development, structure and functions of oral mucosa. In *The Mouth and Perioral Tissues*. (ed. C. Scully), Heinemann Medical, Oxford, 1989
4. Beckett, A. H. and Hossie, R. D. Buccal absorption of drugs. In *Concepts in Biochemical Pharmacology, Part 1*. (eds B. B. Brodie and J. R. Gillette), Springer Verlag, Berlin, pp. 25–46, 1971
5. Schürmann, W. and Turner, P. A membrane model of the human oral mucosa as derived from buccal absorption performance and physicochemical properties of the β-blocking drugs atenolol and propranolol. *Journal of Pharmacy and Pharmacology*, **30**, 137–147, 1978
6. Henry, J. A., Ohashi, K., Wadsworth, J. and Turner, P. Drug recovery following buccal absorption of propranolol. *British Journal of Clinical Pharmacology*, **10**, 61–65, 1980
7. Squier, C. A. and Johnson, N. W. Permeability of oral mucosa. *British Medical Bulletin*, **31**, 169–175, 1975

8. Abrams, J. Pharmacology of nitroglycerin and long-acting nitrates. *American Journal of Cardiology*, **56** (Suppl. 2), 12A–18A, 1985
9. Blumenthal, H. P., Fung, H. L., McNiff, E. F. and Yap, S. K. Plasma nitroglycerin levels after sublingual, oral and topical administration. *British Journal of Clinical Pharmacology*, **4**, 241–242, 1977
10. Morrison, R. A., Wiegand, U.-W., Jähnchen, E., Höhmann, D., Bechtold, H., Meinertz, T. and Fung, H.-L. Isosorbide dinitrate kinetics and dynamics after intravenous, sublingual, and percutaneous dosing in angina. *Clinical Pharmacology and Therapeutics*, **33**, 747–756, 1983
11. Parker, J. O., Vankjoughnett, K. A. and Farrell, B. Nitroglycerin lingual spray: clinical efficacy and dose–response relation. *American Journal of Cardiology*, **57**, 1–5, 1986
12. Haft, J. I. and Litterer, W. E. Chewing nifedipine to rapidly treat hypertension. *Archives of Internal Medicine*, **144**, 2357–2359, 1984
13. McAllister, R. G., Jr. Kinetics and dynamics of nifedipine after oral and sublingual doses. *American Journal of Medicine*, **81** (Suppl. 6A), 2–5, 1986
14. Van Harten, J., Danhof, M., Burggraaf, K., Van Brummelen, P. and Breimer, D. D. Negligible sublingual absorption of nifedipine. *Lancet*, **ii**, 1363–1365, 1987
15. Asthana, O. P., Woodcock, B. G., Wenchel, M., Frömming, K. H., Schwabe, L. and Rietbrock, N. Verapamil disposition and effect on PQ-intervals after buccal, oral and intravenous administration. *Arzneimittel-Forschung*, **34**, 498–502, 1984
16. Bell, M. D. D., Murray, G. R., Mishra, P., Calvey, T. N. and Williams, N. E. Buccal morphine – a new route for analgesia? *Lancet*, **i**, 71–73, 1985
17. Bullingham, R. E. S., McQuay, H. J., Porter, E. J. B., Allen, M. C. and Moore, R. A. Sublingual buprenorphine used postoperatively: ten hour plasma drug concentration analysis. *British Journal of Clinical Pharmacology*, **13**, 665–673, 1982
18. Editorial. Sublingual buprenorphine. *Drug and Therapeutics Bulletin*, **20**, 74–76, 1982
19. Brown, A. S. Absorption of analgesics from the buccal mucous membrane. *Practitioner*, **196**, 125–126, 1966
20. Winsor, T. Plethysmographic comparison of sublingual and intramuscular ergotamine. *Clinical Pharmacology and Therapeutics*, **29**, 94–99, 1981
21. Sutherland, J. M., Hooper, W. D., Eadie, M. J. and Tyrer, J. H. Buccal absorption of ergotamine. *Journal of Neurology, Neurosurgery, and Psychiatry*, **37**, 1116–1120, 1974
22. Ward, A. E. Studies of prochlorperazine as a buccal tablet (Buccastem) and an oral tablet (Stemetil) for the treatment of dizziness, nausea or vomiting in a general practice setting. *British Journal of Clinical Practice*, **42**, 228–232, 1988
23. Burnier, A. M., Martin, P. L., Yen, S. S. C. and Brooks, P. Sublingual absorption of micronized 17β-estradiol. *American Journal of Obstetrics and Gynecology*, **140**, 146–150, 1981
24. Casper, R. F. and Yen, S. S. C. Rapid absorption of micronized estradiol-17β following sublingual administration. *Obstetrics and Gynecology*, **57**, 62–64, 1981
25. Dawood, M. Y., Ylikorkala, O. and Fuchs, F. Plasma oxytocin levels and disappearance rate after buccal Pitocin. *American Journal of Obstetrics and Gynecology*, **138**, 20–24, 1980
26. Ishida, M., Machida, Y., Nambu, N. and Nagai, T. New mucosal dosage form of insulin. *Chemical and Pharmaceutical Bulletin*, **29**, 810–816, 1981

27. Anders, R. and Merkle, H. P. Buccal absorption of protirelin: an effective way to stimulate thyrotropin and prolactin. *Journal of Pharmaceutical Sciences,* **72**, 1481–1483, 1983

Further reading

Meyer, J., Squier, C. A. and Gerson, S. J. *The Structure and Function of Oral Mucosa,* Pergamon Press, Oxford, 1984

Jenkins, G. N. *The Physiology and Biochemistry of the Mouth,* Blackwell Scientific, Oxford, 1978

Sneebny, L. M. (ed.) *The Salivary System,* Wolfe Medical, London, 1987

3

Drug delivery to the respiratory tract

S. J. Farr, I. W. Kellaway and G. Taylor

Introduction

The respiratory tract has long been employed as a route of drug administration, principally to achieve localized drug action rather than for delivery to the systemic system. The morphology of the lung is such that to achieve effective drug deposition it is necessary to control the characteristics of the dosage form, particularly particle size. All devices employed to deliver drugs to the bronchial tree generate an aerosol. This is a relatively stable two-phase system consisting of finely divided condensed matter in a gaseous continuum; the condensed disperse phase may be liquid, solid or a combination of the two and by virtue of the size requirements may be considered as a colloidal dispersion.

For many years, compounds such as benzoin, creosote, eucalyptus, menthol and thymol have been inhaled as vapours arising from hot aqueous dispersions. Although these volatile aromatics do have a mild irritant action, a substantial benefit undoubtedly accrues from the expectorant effect of warm air of high humidity. With the advent of more potent molecules such as the bronchodilators and corticosteroids, more efficient devices have been developed and drug delivery to the lungs is now achieved by three principal types of device: pressurized pack metered-dose inhalers, nebulizers for continuous administration and unit-dose dry powder inhalers

Drug delivery to the nasal mucosa, in addition to the lungs, is an increasingly important route of administration for the achievement of systemic drug levels (see Chapter 1). This chapter reviews the features of respiratory tract morphology and physiology relevant to drug administration, drugs used and their fate, and the disease states treated. Pharmaceutical formulations of these drugs are outlined, together with the design features of the devices employed. Finally, evaluation procedures both *in vitro* and *in vivo* for drug delivery systems are described.

Respiratory tract morphology and physiology

The lung is a specialized tissue with the prime function of gaseous exchange involving oxygen absorption and carbon dioxide and water elimination. Efficient exchange results from a surface area of approximately $70\,m^2$ and an air–blood barrier of between 0.36 and 2.5 μm. It has been estimated that the daily air mass dealt with by the human lung is approximately 13 kg. The lung therefore provides a great potential for toxicity by airborne toxins and, in addition, some substances that are poorly absorbed in the gut are well retained by, and absorbed within, the lung.

For convenience, the respiratory tract (Figure 3.1) is often compartmentalized into the following three regions (Table 3.1):

1. The nasopharyngeal (NP) (or oropharyngeal) compartment, which consists of the nares and mouth and includes the respiratory airways down to the larynx;
2. The tracheobronchial (TB) region, which begins at the larynx and includes the trachea and the ciliated bronchial airways down to the terminal bronchioles;
3. The pulmonary (P) (or functional gaseous exchange) region, which comprises the respiratory bronchioles, alveolar ducts, alveolar sacs, atria and alveoli.

The terms 'upper' and 'lower' respiratory tract are frequently

Table 3.1 Compartmentalization of the respiratory tract*

Compartment	Deposition	Clearance	Pathology
Nasopharyngeal (NP)	Impaction Diffusion Interception Electrostatic	Muciliary Sneezing Blowing	Inflammation Ulceration Cancer
Tracheobronchial (TB)	Impaction Sedimentation Diffusion Interception	Mucociliary (hours) Coughing	Bronchospasm Obstruction Cancer
Pulmonary (P)	Sedimentation Diffusion Interception	Solubilization Phagocytosis Interstitial (hours to years)	Inflammation Oedema Emphysema Fibrosis Cancer

* As reported by the Task Group on Lung Dynamics of the International Commission on Radiological Protection[1].

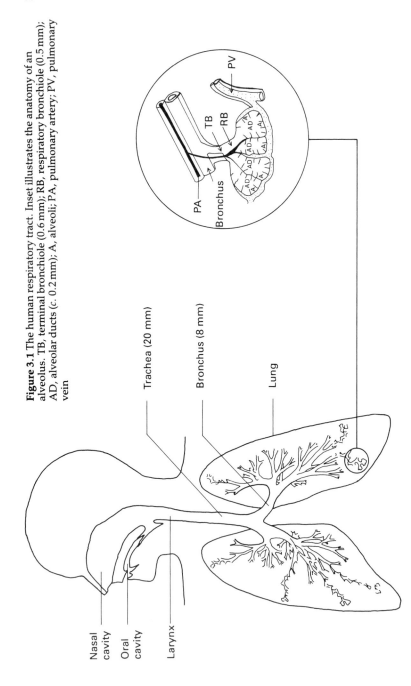

Figure 3.1 The human respiratory tract. Inset illustrates the anatomy of an alveolus. TB, terminal bronchiole (0.6 mm); RB, respiratory bronchiole (0.5 mm); AD, alveolar ducts (c. 0.2 mm); A, alveoli; PA, pulmonary artery; PV, pulmonary vein

encountered and correspond to the NP together with the trachea, and the P plus bronchial regions, respectively.

The NP compartment can entrap larger particles, the inertia of which causes impaction in the nasal passages or entrapment by nasal hairs. Clearance is believed to occur either by particle dissolution and distribution into blood or, for less soluble materials, physical clearance by mucociliary transport with subsequent swallowing. The posterior region of the nose is subject to mucociliary clearance, whereas particles deposited in the anterior region will be cleared only by such actions as wiping, sneezing or nose blowing.

A relatively small fraction of all inhaled particles will deposit in the TB region. TB deposition may occur by a variety of mechanisms but principally by inertial impaction, sedimentation and Brownian diffusion – the latter restricted to submicron particles. Mouth breathing of aerosols – the normal route of pulmonary delivery of medicinal agents – bypasses the nasal removal of large particulates, which therefore are deposited in the throat and parts of the TB region. The 'mucociliary escalator' ensures rapid (within hours) removal of insoluble deposited particles; soluble particles dissolve and may enter the bloodstream. Mucus is removed by the cilia at a rate which increases as the diameter of the airways increases. This, in conjunction with the tendency towards deeper penetration of the lung for smaller particles, ensures that larger particles are cleared more rapidly. It is for this reason that particle clearance kinetics from this compartment cannot be described by a single rate, although estimates of clearance half-time of 0.5, 2.5 and 5 h have been quoted for the larger, intermediate and finer airways respectively.

For particles to deposit in the deepest compartment (the P region), successful penetration beyond the NP and TB regions must occur, with subsequent retention on the pulmonary surfaces as a result of settling, diffusion and interception processes (the relative contribution being, to a large extent, governed by particle size)[2]. The residual volume (approximately 1.2 l air) ensures that for some particles the time necessary to achieve deposition may be considerably longer than a single breathing cycle and, in some instances, may be minutes rather than seconds. Several mechanisms ensure clearance from this region and include dissolution with absorption, phagocytosis of particles by macrophages with translocation to the ciliated airways, lymphatic uptake of particles and the possibility of direct passage of particles into the bloodstream.

These three compartments were adopted by the ICRP Task Group examining the relationship between fraction deposited and particle aerodynamic diameter[1], and subsequently applied to the mouth breathing of monodispersed aerosols (Figure 3.2). These theoretical profiles are in reasonable agreement with experimentally determined curves (Figure 3.3).

Cells and tissues of the respiratory tract

The ultrastructure of the trachea and large bronchi consists of a variety of cells including ciliated and goblet cells, which predominate, and serous, basal, brush, undifferentiated, Clara and Kulchitsky cells[5]. In the bronchioles, ciliated cells are dominant and Clara cells progressively increase distally along the airways. Goblet cells and serous cells also decrease distally and are absent in terminal bronchioles. Undifferentiated brush, basal and Kulchitsky cells are an uncommon occurrence. The cells and tissues which have an important role in drug

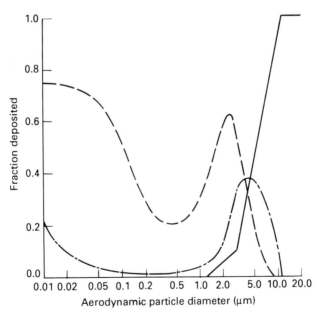

Figure 3.2 Theoretical deposition of monodisperse aerosols inhaled by healthy human adults in the 'head' (——), tracheobronchial (— – — –) and pulmonary (– – – –) regions of the respiratory tract during normal mouth breathing. (Adapted from reference 3)

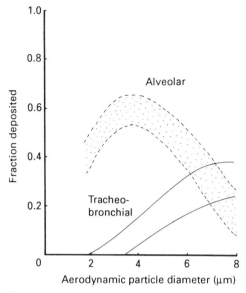

Figure 3.3 Particle diameter dependence of alveolar and tracheobronchial deposition for mouth breathing. Tidal volume 1 l, breathing frequency 7.5/min, mean flow rate 250 cm^3/s, inspiration/expiration times 4 s each. (Adapted from reference 4)

deposition and clearance are the ciliated mucosae and the alveoli.

Ciliated mucosa

Ciliated mucosal tissue lines the rear portion of the nose, the larynx and the tracheobronchial tree. The cilia are hair-like projections which beat in a coordinated fashion to move the overlying mucus blanket in a direction towards the throat, where the mucus is swallowed. The mucus, primarily an acid glycoprotein, is produced from goblet cells and sub-mucosal glands which are interspersed with the ciliated cells; all cell types are attached to the basement membrane. Mucus is a viscoelastic, tacky fluid which is responsible in conjunction with the cilia for the removal of particulates from the tracheobronchial regions. The efficiency of the 'mucociliary escalator' depends on the quantity and quality of mucus and the number and synchronization of the cilia. Drugs that can alter the viscoelastic properties of mucus range from mucolytics such as N-acetylcysteine, which reduce the viscosity and elasticity, to mucospicics such as the tetracyclines, which enhance both the viscous and elastic nature of the mucus gel. There appears to be a range of mucus elasticity within which cilia can effect transport.

Viral and bacterial infections can lead to changes in both the quantity and quality of the mucus and, in more severe cases, clearance is possible only through the action of coughing or sneezing.

Alveoli

The alveoli are polyhedral structures, generally <300 μm in diameter, surrounded by thin-walled epithelial cells on all but one side which is open to the atmosphere. The epithelial cells are of several types: Type I are thin cells, overlying a basement membrane c. 20–40 nm thick. A much thicker but smaller cell (Type II) has a surface covered with microvilli, which greatly increase the surface area in contact with the airstream. These cells produce and secrete 'lung surfactant', which is composed of lipid-rich lipoproteins (85–90% w/w lipid). The lipid composition is dominated by phosphatidylcholines, with dipalmitoyl phosphatidylcholine in unusually high percentages. This mixture leads to the generation of low, stable surface tensions, preventing collapse of the lung. Proteins present include serum albumin, together with 10 and 35 kDa non-serum proteins. The latter allow the rapid formation of phospholipid surface films in the alveoli. Respiratory distress syndrome is an example of a disease state related to abnormalities in lung surfactants. Type III, or alveolar brush cells, overlie the alveolar basement membrane and protrude into the airspace with their large microvilli. Other cell types include interstitial cells and macrophages. The alveolar macrophages are mobile, nucleated cells which surround and endocytose small particles; the function of maintaining sterility by engulfing and killing microorganisms, together with 'dust collecting', has been ascribed to these cells. Both positive and negative chemotactic responses have been demonstrated by alveolar macrophages; certain dusts, e.g. coal, asbestos and silica, may be cytotoxic to macrophages, and an upper limit of 8 μm has been suggested for phagocytic uptake.

Diseases of the lung

Respiratory infections

The volume of air handled by the lung each day is in excess of 10 000 l and the respiratory system is prone to assault by a variety of microbes, allergens and toxins. As a consequence it is not surprising that respiratory infections by bacteria and viruses are common. A large number of pathogenic bacteria, viruses and fungi are potential causes of inflammation of the lungs (pneumonia), although infection with *Streptococcus pneumoniae* (the pneumococcus) is commonly encountered. The usual treatment of pneumonia involves chemotherapy with one of the penicillins or co-trimoxazole given systemically by either the oral or the parenteral route. Local administration of antibacterials to the lungs by inhalation is occasionally performed, although in general it does not offer any advantages over the systemic route and is not routinely practised[6]. However, an exception is the use of pentamidine isethionate for the treatment of *Pneumocystis carinii* pneumonia. In this life-threatening respiratory disease of severely immunocompromised patients (including those with AIDS), the infection resides extracellularly in the alveolar space; the use of nebulizers to target drug to the appropriate region in the lung results in improved efficacy and a substantial reduction in the dose-related extrapulmonary toxicity associated with intravenous therapy (see Chapter 5).

Bronchial asthma

Many different types of particle suspended in the atmosphere are capable of stimulating the production of antibodies when inhaled. This may result in the development of a number of allergic diseases of the respiratory system, including bronchial asthma, allergic alveolitis and allergic rhinitis. Bronchial asthma results from a narrowing of the bronchi by muscle spasm, mucosal swelling or tenacious mucus secretion. Asthma occurs in a number of different forms, some of which have a demonstrable allergic aetiology (extrinsic asthma), whereas others appear to be reactions to infection, psychological factors or non-specific physical and chemical stimuli (intrinsic asthma). The acute asthmatic attack is of sudden onset, occurring at any time, day or night, and is manifest primarily as difficulty in forcing air out of the narrowed airways resulting in wheezing sounds, breathlessness and discomfort during breathing. The attacks may end abruptly in less than an hour or may persist for several days. An asthmatic attack which persists for more than a few hours may progress to severe acute asthma (status asthmaticus) in which the smaller bronchi become completely obstructed, leading to a life-threatening situation of alveolar hypoventilation, arterial hypoxaemia, tachycardia and central cyanosis and ultimately culminating in cardiac arrest.

In chronic asthma, wheeze is almost continuously present together with breathlessness on exertion; however, the sudden onset of attacks is less pronounced. Because the removal of mucus (and entrapped microbes) is impaired in chronic asthmatics, respiratory infections commonly recur in these individuals and the symptoms of chronic bronchitis and emphysema may also be present. Extrinsic asthma is fairly common in atopic individuals, who readily form IgE antibodies to frequently encountered allergens and who often suffer from hay fever and allergic dermatitis. It is usually first manifest in children or young adults, and the allergens commonly involved derive from pollen, mites in house dust, animal dander, foods and drugs. The inhaled allergen reacts with IgE on sensitized mast cells, causing the release of a number of factors including histamine, bradykinin and slow-reacting substance A (SRS-A), which either directly or indirectly cause bronchoconstriction and an inflammatory response.

Occupational respiratory diseases

Extrinsic allergic alveolitis encompasses a number of disease states including farmer's lung, pigeon-fancier's lung and maltworker's lung, and results from the inhalation of certain types of organic dust such as *Microspora* from mouldy hay, avian excreta, and *Aspergillus* from malting barley. The main feature of these diseases is a widespread allergic reaction in the alveoli and interstitium (unlike extrinsic asthma, where the allergic reaction occurs in the bronchi).

The occupational inhalation of cotton dust may lead to mill fever, weaver's cough and byssinosis, which have features in common with allergic alveolitis and asthma. Pneumoconiosis results from the prolonged inhalation of various mineral dusts such as coal dust (coalworker's pneumoconiosis), silica (silicosis) and asbestos (asbestosis); its various forms are marked by pulmonary fibrosis, which in part is attributable to overburdening of the macrophages which remove dust particles deposited in the alveolar regions of the lungs[7].

Chronic bronchitis and emphysema

Chronic bronchitis and emphysema often occur together and are frequent complications of other disease states such as chronic asthma and pneumoconiosis. Airflow impedance is common to both chronic bronchitis and emphysema and terms such as 'chronic obstructive airways disease' are used to describe these disease states; however, they have distinct pathological features. The principal feature of chronic bronchitis appears to be overproduction of mucus by the goblet cells, which enlarge and eventually replace the ciliated epithelial cells. This combination of events leads to distortion and obstruction of the smaller airways. Chronic bronchitis is common in patients having long-term exposure to irritants of bronchial mucosa such as tobacco smoke, dust, fumes and other atmospheric pollutants. Other factors involved in precipitating the disease may be infection, fog and sudden changes in temperature. Emphysema is characterized by overdistension of the respiratory bronchioles and alveoli caused by trapped air or destruction of their walls. Air becomes trapped in emphysematous areas due to distortion or partial obstruction of airways, which allows air to enter these regions more readily than it can be exhaled. The distension caused by emphysema tends to obstruct neighbouring regions, thus spreading the area of damage. Emphysema is a common complication of chronic bronchitis and asthma.

Chemotherapy of respiratory diseases

Drug administration

The most obvious method of achieving therapeutic concentrations of a drug at a receptor site within the lung is to administer the drug by inhalation as an aerosol using a pressurized pack, nebulizer or dry powder inhaler. However, most drugs acting on the lung may also reach their sites of action from the systemic circulation and are effective when administered by parenteral or oral routes. Local administration of drugs rapidly produces relatively high concentrations of drug close to the site of action and may reduce side-effects associated with high concentrations of drug in the systemic circulation: for example, corticosteroids are administered by the inhalation route in asthma to circumvent adverse systemic glucocorticoid side-effects. A further advantage of the inhalational route is that any first-pass metabolism or malabsorption seen after oral dosing will be avoided. The inhalational route does, however, have its limitations: these are the size of dose that may be administered, the degree of expertise required to self-administer doses reproducibly and its inconvenience compared with the oral route. Many drugs that act on the lung are therefore administered orally, although the daily dose may be 10–20 times greater than the inhaled dose and 100 times the dose actually deposited in the lung. A possible method of targeting drugs to the lung from the systemic circulation is to link the drug to a colloidal carrier of a suitable size, so that after intravenous administration the carrier becomes entrapped within the capillary bed of the pulmonary circulation, whereupon it leaches the drug[8].

In addition to simple partitioning between the systemic circulation and lung tissues, many xenobiotics are taken up by, and show a high degree of accumulation in, lung parenchyma. Organic bases such as chlorpromazine, imipramine, morphine, propranolol and paraquat accumulate by simple diffusion from the systemic circulation followed by binding to lung tissues[9], resulting in extensive accumulation (propranolol has been reported to achieve a lung tissue/plasma concentration ratio of 250). Accumulation of such compounds is also likely to occur if they are administered by inhalation to the lung.

Bronchodilators

A number of different types of drug including bronchodilators, anti-inflammatory agents and mast cell-stabilizing agents, administered locally or systemically, are used in the chemotherapy of asthma[10]. The commonly used bronchodilators include a variety of adrenoceptor stimulants, anticholinergics and xanthines. Adrenoceptor stimulants act via receptors located on smooth muscle cells in the airway walls, causing an increase in intracellular c-AMP which results in relaxation of the smooth muscle fibres and resultant bronchodilation. However, in addition to stimulation of adrenergic receptors in the airways, non-selective catecholamines such as adrenaline and isoprenaline stimulate cardiac receptors and may elicit side-effects including tachycardia and arrhythmias. Selective β_2-adrenoceptor agonists including salbutamol, salmeterol, fenoterol, isoetharine, pirbuterol, rimiterol and terbutaline are generally free of cardiac side-effects and are commonly used in treating asthmatic attacks. These drugs are preferentially given by inhalation of aerosol from a pressurized pack, nebulizer or dry powder inhaler, because inhalation is less likely to produce side-effects such as anxiety and tremor which can occur after oral dosing. Airflow obstruction in chronic bronchitis and emphysema is less reversible than in asthma, and β_2-adrenoceptor agonists are generally less useful in the therapy of these disease states.

Atropine and ipratropium are effective anticholinergic bronchodilators that tend to be administered by inhalation (in combination with other bronchodilators) in the chemotherapy of asthma. Additionally, ipratropium is indicated for the relief of bronchoconstriction in chronic bronchitis, where it may be more effective than β_2-adrenoceptor agonists. Xanthines such as theophylline and aminophylline produce bronchodilation by a number of mechanisms, including stimulation of endogenous catecholamines and increasing intracellular c-AMP by an inhibition of phosphodiesterase. Xanthines are usually administered as oral sustained-release dosage forms and may have advantages over β_2-adrenoceptor agonists in preventing nocturnal asthma and early-morning wheezing. Aminophylline, salbutamol and terbutaline are also given parenterally in the treatment of severe acute asthma.

Corticosteroids

In addition to bronchodilators, which have an immediate effect on airways obstruction, a number of other drugs are used in the suppression and prophylaxis of asthma, particularly chronic asthma. Corticosteroids are often given for stabilization of frequently occurring asthmatic attacks, especially in adults. When given in combination with β_2-adrenoceptor agonists, corticosteroids help to reduce the frequency of dosing of these drugs. They are of little value in the therapy of chronic bronchitis or emphysema. Corticosteroids such as beclomethasone, betamethasone and budesonide relieve airflow obstruction indirectly, by reducing allergic reactions and suppressing bronchial mucosal inflammatory reactions, thus reducing bronchial hyperreactivity, oedema and hypersecretion of mucus. Their mode of action is not fully understood but involves preventing the release from cell membranes of phospholipids, which are converted to a number of inflammatory mediators including leukotrienes and prostaglandins. In cases of severe bronchospasm and extrinsic allergic alveolitis, short high-dose courses of oral corticosteroids are used; intractable chronic asthma may require continuous oral corticosteroid therapy. Intravenous corticosteroids are also used in the emergency treatment of severe acute asthma.

Prophylactics

A few drugs, including sodium cromoglycate, ketotifen and nedocromil, are used in the prophylaxis of asthma and other reversible obstructive airways diseases. These drugs reduce the incidence of asthmatic attacks and help to reduce doses of concurrently administered bronchodilators and corticosteroids. Sodium cromoglycate is especially of value in children with extrinsic and exercise-induced asthma (which is not uncommon in atopic children), and acts by stabilizing sensitized mast cells in the airway walls, thereby inhibiting the release of mediators of the allergic reaction. Sodium cromoglycate is administered by inhalation from a dry powder inhaler, pressurized pack or nebulizer; it is not given systemically. Ketotifen acts in a similar manner to sodium cromoglycate but is currently given only by the oral route. The anti-inflammatory agent nedocromil acts by inhibiting the release of inflammatory mediators from a variety of cell types located in the lumen and mucosa of the airways; it is currently used only in adults and is administered by inhalation.

Mucolytics

Tenacious mucus is a common symptom in chronic bronchitis and a number of other respiratory disease states[11]. However, the number of mucolytics currently in use is small. Mucolytics such as N-acetylcysteine and tyloxapol have been given by inhalation (or, less frequently, orally) to reduce sputum viscosity in chronic bronchitis and cystic fibrosis.

Drugs used in minor respiratory disorders

A wide variety of drugs, such as cough suppressants, expectorants, demulcents and decongestants, are used in the treatment of minor respiratory disorders and are almost invariably given orally. Despite their widespread use the value of these agents in the treatment of cough and congestion is contentious. The commonly used cough suppressants include opiates and related compounds such as codeine, pholcodine and papaverine; diamorphine and methadone are more potent but generally are reserved for care of the terminally ill. These drugs are thought to act centrally, on the cough centre, rather than locally. Demulcents, including glycerol, syrup and sorbitol, may help to sooth dry irritating coughs by a topical effect, although they are likely to be effective only when the site of irritation is located above the level of the epiglottis. Expectorants, by definition, act by promoting expulsion of sputum; however, there is little evidence that any of the commonly used agents such as ammonium chloride, guaiphenesin and ipecacuanha are effective expectorants. Their mode of action is not local but may lie in stimulation of the cough reflex. Sympatho-mimetic agents such as ephedrine, phenylpropanolamine and pseudoephedrine, in addition to antihistamines such as brompheniramine, diphenhydramine, promethazine and tripro-lidine, are claimed to reduce congestion; the more sedating antihistamines may also act as antitussives.

Fate of compounds administered to the respiratory tract

Absorption

Most drugs are administered to the respiratory tract in order to produce a local effect and to minimize side-effects that may be associated with giving the drug systemically. However, the extensive surface area of the lung, which is almost as large as that of the small intestine, combined with a thin epithelial membrane and a rich blood supply, make the lung a possible major route for the entry of foreign compounds into the systemic circulation. The most common use of the lungs as a delivery route for systemically acting compounds is in gaseous anaesthesia and oxygen therapy. Assessing the absorption of non-volatile compounds from the lung has proved difficult in many instances because administration by aerosols results in only 5–20% of the administered dose being deposited in the lung itself, with a significant proportion of the remainder reaching the gastrointestinal tract. Direct instillation into the trachea or bronchi has been routinely used in animal studies, but the pattern of deposition using this technique may not be the same as that following administration by aerosol. It is difficult to assess the permeabilities of the tracheobronchial and pulmonary epithelia *in vivo* because of the elaborate structure of the lung, although it is generally accepted that absorption occurs more rapidly through the thinner epithelial membranes of the pulmonary region.

The fate of foreign compounds within the lung depends largely upon their solubility and lipophilicity. Depending upon their size, insoluble particles such as dusts and microbes either become entrapped in the mucus secretions, or reach the pulmonary regions where they are rapidly endocytosed by alveolar macrophages. Endocytosed particles inside the alveolar macrophages are transferred to the mucociliary escalator for removal; this is a major defence mechanism of the lung and ensures that the alveoli remain sterile despite the inhalation of appreciable numbers of microbes. Endocytosis of particles in the alveolar regions also occurs by cells other than macrophages, and the removal of certain large, very poorly soluble particles may take a number of years.

Compounds which dissolve in pulmonary surfactant are absorbed from the lung by a number of different processes, including active transport and passive diffusion through both aqueous pores and lipoidal regions of the epithelial membranes. Many compounds are absorbed more rapidly from the lung than from the small intestine. Furthermore, some compounds are absorbed much more efficiently from the lung: for example, <5% of the anti-asthmatic drug sodium cromoglycate is absorbed from the gastrointestinal tract, whereas it is well absorbed from the lung. As the epithelial membranes of the lung are principally lipoidal, a rapid uptake of both volatile and non-volatile lipophilic compounds occurs, and a rich blood supply ensures that compounds are then rapidly transferred to the systemic circulation. Volatile substances such as lipophilic gaseous anaesthetics are absorbed very rapidly from the lung. The rate of absorption of these compounds tends to increase with increasing lipophilicity up to the point where solubility in blood becomes the rate-limiting factor. Similarly, the absorption of non-volatile lipophilic compounds tends to increase with increasing lipophilicity until solubility in either the lung surfactant or blood becomes rate limiting. Absorption of these compounds generally occurs by a non-saturable passive diffusion process.

The absorption of hydrophilic compounds is generally slower than that of lipophilic compounds. In addition to the lipoidal regions, lung epithelium has aqueous pores of various sizes. Passage through the aqueous pores appears to be the principal route of absorption for hydrophilic compounds and the rate of absorption tends to decrease with increasing molecular weight. Certain hydrophilic compounds that are too large to pass through aqueous pores in the gastrointestinal tract are well absorbed through the lung, for example sodium cromoglycate and gentamicin. Additionally, at least two carrier-mediated transport systems exist for lung absorption: one transports organic anions such as sodium cromoglycate and phenol red; the other transports certain amino acids. Sodium cromoglycate is absorbed from the rat lung by both active transport and passive diffusion.

Metabolism

As the lungs are similar to the gastrointestinal tract in being a major route of entry for foreign compounds, detoxication may be an important defence mechanism. Most of the xenobiotic-metabolizing systems present in liver are also present in lung, but although the content of most enzymes in the lung is less than that of liver, the blood flow normalized for tissue weight is approximately tenfold higher in the lung and therefore can make a significant contribution to metabolic clearance of compounds within the systemic circulation [12]. The lung has an important role in the metabolism of endogenous compounds such as serotonin, bradykinin, noradrenaline, steroids and in the conversion of angiotensin I to angiotensin II. The lung is capable both of Phase I oxidation, reduction and hydrolysis reactions involving cytochrome P-450, amine oxidase, epoxide hydrolase, reductases and esterases, and also of Phase II conjugation reactions involving glucuronyl transferase, sulpho-transferase, N-acetyltransferase, methyltransferases and glutathione S-transferase.

The metabolism of foreign compounds administered to the lungs is difficult to quantify because up to 40 different types of cell may exist in the lung, each having a different spectrum of metabolic activity. The situation is further complicated as no single cell species is predominant and accessibility of administered compounds to the metabolically important cells is usually unknown. Lung cytochrome P-450-dependent mixed function oxidase activity tends to be concentrated in the bronchiolar and alveolar epithelial cells, although trachea and bronchi have been shown to metabolize compounds such as benzpyrene. The non-ciliated bronchiolar epithelial (Clara) cells and alveolar Type II cells appear to be the most important for the metabolism of xenobiotics. Non-cytochrome P-450-dependent systems such as amine oxidase, glutathione S-transferase and glucuronyl transferase are also present in these two cell types. Alveolar macrophages are reported to contain esterases, phospholipases, proteases and β-glucuronidase. Additionally, human alveolar macrophages show aryl hydrocarbon hydroxylase activity, which appears to be induced in smokers.

Enzyme systems that are of particular importance within the lung include methyltransferases, reductases and epoxide hydro-lase. Although methylation is not generally one of the most important metabolic reactions within the body, the lung has an unusually high capacity for this biotransformation. Drugs, such as isoprenaline and isoetharine, that resemble endogenous catecholamines are substrates for catechol O-methyltransferase. It has been noted that intrabronchial administration of isoprenaline results in much higher concentrations of the O-methyl metabolite than those following intravenous administration, whereas oral administration results primarily in the formation of the sulphate conjugate. Other methyltransferases are responsible for the N-methylation of desmethylimipramine, nortriptyline and aniline within the lung. Reductases may be responsible for the generation of free radicals from pulmonary toxins such as paraquat and mitomycin C, which react with oxygen to regenerate parent drug and form superoxide. Epoxide hydrolase functions to convert reactive epoxides formed by the cytochrome P-450 mixed function oxidase system to dihydrodiols. The activities of this enzyme are fairly low in the lung and reportedly absent from Type II alveolar cells; the lung may therefore be particularly susceptible to damage by substrates that form epoxides. Thus, although metabolic processes largely result in detoxication, in certain cases toxic metabolites may be formed. Indeed, toxic metabolites, including epoxides from benzpyrene and naphthalene and free radicals from paraquat and carbon tetrachloride, have been identified within the lung.

Generation of therapeutic aerosols

Particle size considerations

An important feature in the design of a therapeutic aerosol is that for maximum efficacy the particles/droplets containing the drug need to be generated as a size that will deposit in the lower regions of the lung when inhaled, i.e. 2–5 μm in diameter. The pharmaceutical formulator, therefore, is concerned not only with the design of a device that ensures product stability from the time of manufacture to its subsequent use, but also one that is capable of generating an aerosol cloud that can be inhaled in a convenient manner by the patient.

The size of particles or droplets in an aerosol is expressed in terms of aerodynamic diameter, defined as the diameter of a spherical particle with unit density that settles at the same rate as the particle being described. Thus in the simplest case, when the particles being described are spherical (as is assumed to be the case with therapeutic aerosols) with a diameter d and a density ρ, the aerodynamic diameter, d_a, is given by the relation:

$$d_a = d \sqrt{\rho/\rho_o}$$

where ρ_o is unit density ($1\,kg/m^3$).

The aerodynamic diameter dividing the size distribution into two halves is termed the mass median aerodynamic diameter (MMAD) and this, together with the geometric standard deviation (σ_g), are used to describe adequately the range of sizes observed within an aerosol distribution. In a log-normal distribution, which is prevalent in aerosol systems, σ_g is a measure of the polydispersity of the aerosol and is the ratio of the diameter of the particle at 84.2% on the cumulative frequency curve to the median diameter. An ideal monodisperse population (i.e. where the particles making up the aerosol are all the same size) would have a σ_g of 1, but in practice aerosols with σ_g <1.22 are described as monodisperse and >1.22 as polydisperse (or heterodisperse).

Devices for drug administration to the lung

Three important categories of aerosol generator are used in inhalation therapy [13]:

1. Pressurized pack (metered-dose) inhaler;
2. Nebulizer;
3. Unit-dose dry powder inhaler.

Pressurized pack

Pressurized packs may be defined as 'self-contained sprayable products in which the propellant force is a liquefied or compressed gas'. They were introduced in inhalation therapy over 20 years ago and remain the major device used by domiciliary patients [10, 14].

The unit consists of a container (typically 10 ml volume) hermetically sealed by means of a metering valve (Figure 3.4). The containers, which must be chemically inert, are normally composed of aluminium and fabricated by extrusion to avoid the presence of seams. As a result, the containers are mechanically strong and can withstand internal pressures well in excess of 400 kPa. Glass containers protected with a plastic outer casing to protect against accidental shattering are an alternative, but can be employed only for units of lower internal pressure.

Most drugs delivered to the lung exhibit low solubility in the liquid propellants used and therefore are frequently formulated as suspensions of micronized drug particles. These possess significant surface energy and require the addition of a low concentration of surfactant (sorbitan esters, lecithin, oleic acid) to improve the suspension's stability. Such excipients are also

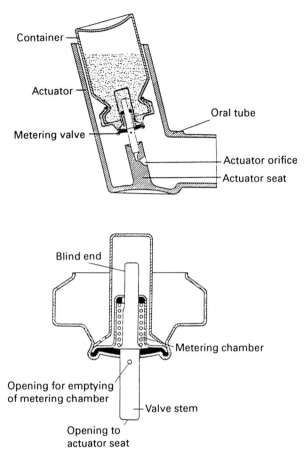

Figure 3.4 Diagram of a metered dose inhaler and metering valve. (Reproduced from reference 14, with permission)

necessary to lubricate the metering valve assembly to ensure accurate and reproducible operation. Alternatively, the drug substance may be dissolved in the liquid propellant by the addition of a suitable cosolvent, typically large amounts of ethanol.

The propellant blend consists of a mixture of two or three chlorofluorocarbons, identified by a numbering system. Propellant 11, a liquid at room temperature, is contained in all commercially available suspension-type pressurized packs at a level of at least 25%. Propellant 12 alone, or in combination with

Propellant 114 (both having sub-zero boiling points), is further incorporated to generate the required vapour pressure. Thus a wide variety of internal vapour pressures may be obtained (in accordance with Raoult's law) although, in practice, blends are selected with vapour pressures equivalent to 350–450 kPa.

A dose from a pressurized pack is actuated by depression of an actuator fitted on to the metering valve. When the valve is opened, the internal pressure within the container forces a metered volume of the liquid mixture out through the actuator orifice. Typical volumes range from 25 to 100 μl. In response to a reduction of pressure to atmospheric, a proportion of the liquid propellant immediately evaporates ('flashes'). This serves to disrupt the emerging product into a spray of droplets. The initial velocity of the droplets, propelled by the sudden release of the high vapour pressure within the pressurized pack, is high (30 m/s) although deceleration quickly occurs owing to air resistance. The speed of flashing is so rapid that the system behaves adiabatically, resulting in the remaining liquid propellant becoming supercooled. As a result, further evaporation proceeds at a much slower rate and, dependent on the rate, energy is acquired from the surrounding atmosphere.

Using the technique of laser light diffraction, the continuous change in aerosol size caused by propellant evaporation can be monitored. Mean droplet size immediately upon actuation can be as large as 36 μm, which reduces to c. 12 μm at a distance of 10–25 cm away from the mouthpiece opening. Mass median diameter of the emitted spray approaches the original size of the drug crystals only after c. 5 s following actuation. Evaporation is even further retarded by the presence of cosolvents, such as ethanol, with high boiling points; as a result, solution-type aerosols are generally less efficient than suspension aerosols at delivering a therapeutic dose.

Lung deposition of aerosols released from the suspension systems have been assessed following substitution of the micronized drug crystals with ^{99m}Tc-labelled Teflon particles of similar size or by recrystallizing the drug in the presence of ^{99m}Tc. After inhalation, the relative amounts of aerosol depositing in the lungs and oropharynx and the proportion that fails to leave the adaptor are evaluated, using gamma scintigraphy. Such studies frequently show that <10% of the dose reaches the lungs of patients, most of the remainder (>80%) depositing in the oropharynx. Optimization of the inhalation manoeuvre by inspiring slowly with breath-holding for 10 s increases the dose delivered to the lung to only c. 14%.

In recent years the advent of a spacer or extension tube placed between the actuator and the patient's mouth has further improved lung delivery, but high losses still remain. These devices serve as a reservoir into which aerosol doses can be fired, thus affording further opportunity for propellant evaporation and a reduction in velocity of the droplets. They are considered to be of particular importance for those patients who experience problems in the coordination of actuation and inspiration.

Nebulizers

Nebulizers are essentially devices capable of converting an aqueous solution or micronized suspension of drug into an aerosol[15]. Dispersion can be effected by one of two means: by a high-velocity airstream or by ultrasonic energy. Two classes of nebulizer, the air-jet and the ultrasonic, are therefore available.

Air-jet nebulizers

These operate by passing compressed air over the open end of a narrow capillary tube immersed in a liquid reservoir (Figure 3.5). A region of negative pressure (Venturi effect) located above the capillary tube causes liquid to be drawn from the reservoir and converted into a polydisperse aerosol by the high shearing action of the airflow. Larger droplets will impact on the various baffle arrangements and other internal surfaces, and subsequently return to the reservoir. The remaining smaller respirable droplets pass out of the device with the airstream and are inhaled by the patient through a mouthpiece or face-mask.

Currently, over 20 such nebulizers are commercially available with a variety of operating conditions to ensure optimum output and aerosol size distribution. The most common source of compressed gas is from an air or oxygen cylinder, thereby limiting the portability of these devices; they are therefore used far more in hospitals than in the domiciliary environment. The development of cheaper, efficient and compact air compressors should enhance their popularity in places other than hospitals.

Ultrasonic nebulizers

Ultrasonic nebulizers utilize a rapidly oscillating piezoelectric crystal that directs high-frequency waves through a reservoir of drug solution. The result is the production of a dense aerosol plume which is inhaled by the patient. Such units are easily

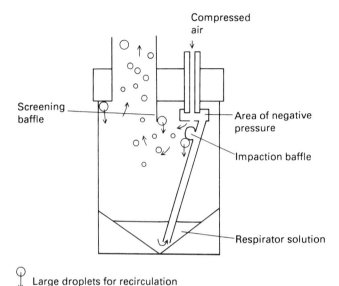

Figure 3.5 Principles of operation of an air-jet nebulizer

portable, rendering their use particularly attractive in the domiciliary environment. However, they are generally expensive and considered to be less robust than air-jet nebulizers.

Formulation aspects of nebulizers

Wherever possible, drugs intended for delivery to the lungs by nebulization are formulated as aqueous solutions. Usually this can be achieved by selection of an appropriate salt and pH to obtain the desired concentration. In certain cases, a cosolvent may be included. Ethanol and/or propylene glycol have been used but will influence both surface tension and viscosity of the solvent system; in turn, these will influence aerosol output and droplet size emitted by the nebulizer.

For drugs of particularly low aqueous solubility, micellar solubilization may be possible by inclusion of surfactants above their critical micelle concentration. For practically insoluble drugs, a micronized suspension stabilized by the addition of surfactants can be employed. Nebulizer solutions may be presented as concentrated solutions from which aliquots are taken and suitably diluted before use. In order to maintain product stability, preservatives, such as benzalkonium chloride, and antoxidants (e.g. sulphites) are included in the formulation. Both excipient types have been implicated with paradoxical bronchospasm[16]; their inclusion may therefore be prohibited in the future. The tendency now is for nebulizer solutions to be presented as small unit-dose solutions that are isotonic and free from any preservative or antoxidant.

Several problems have come to light with nebulizer use. One is that different designs produce different particle sizes of droplets. This, as stated above, is one of the crucial factors affecting deposition; it can be influenced not only by the type of nebulizer, but also may be dependent on correct use by the patient. Microbial contamination of hospital nebulizers has been reported, 20% of the isolates being potentially pathogenic[17]; whereas some authors have found no contamination of the solutions[17], others have[18]. In view of the problem with paradoxical bronchoconstriction attributable to preservatives, it has been suggested that manufacturers should supply unit-dose vials of sterile nebulizer solutions in future[19]. Another potential source of problems is the combination of solutions for inhalation: Ventolin, Bricanyl and Berotec may be mixed with Atrovent (ipratroprium) or with atropine methonitrate solution, but Becotide must not be mixed with other drugs (see Table 3.2).

Table 3.2 Combination of nebulizer solutions*

Permissible combinations†

Ventolin ⎫
Bricanyl ⎬ may be mixed with ⎰ Atrovent
Berotec ⎭   ⎱ Atropine methonitrate solution

Intal may be given sequentially after any of the above without rinsing the nebulizer

Prohibited combinations

Becotide should not be mixed with other drugs.
Antibiotics should never be mixed with other nebulizer solutions or with each other, although colomycin has been dissolved with gentamicin injection and used successfully.

* From reference 20.
† As a guide only.

Dry powder inhalers

Powder inhalers (e.g. Spinhaler*, Rotahalert) are breath-activated systems designed to deliver a set dose of micronized drug on an airstream. A hard gelatin capsule containing the drug is located in a specially engineered tubular plastic device, which can be manipulated to allow discharge of the capsule's contents into the airstream as the patient inhales.

Depending on the dose level contained within the capsule, lactose may be included as a diluent. As the patient inhales, mechanical deaggregation of the powder into single or small aggregates of drug alone is claimed to occur. The energy level required for deaggregation is high and can be achieved only following rapid inhalation by the patient, encouraging inertial impaction of a significant portion of the dose at the back of the throat. Dry powder inhalers, therefore, tend to be even less efficient at delivering therapeutic aerosols to the lung than pressurized packs but, because of the higher doses employed, give rise to equivalent therapeutic effect. Their distinct advantage lies with patients (particularly children) who are unable to overcome the coordination of actuation and inhalation that is essential with the pressurized systems.

Recently, new powder inhaler systems for the administration of drugs to the airways have been introduced. Each is a multidose unit developed to improve ease of use and acceptability among patients. The Diskhalert is designed for use with specially manufactured discs containing salbutamol sulphate (Ventodiskt) or beclomethasone dipropionate (Beco-diskt). A disc, containing eight doses of the drug in separate blisters, is inserted into the inhalation device, which is manipulated to pierce the upper and lower surfaces of one of the blisters with a needle (Figure 3.6). As the patient inhales through the device, the contents of the blister are entrained into the airstream and a percentage is delivered to the lung. The next time that the device is primed, the disc rotates to expose another drug-containing blister to the piercing needle tip.

The Turbuhaler‡ is a unit capable of delivering 200 × 1 mg doses of terbutaline sulphate without the use of any carrier compound. It can be operated simply and is claimed to function at even low inspiratory flow rates, such as those present during acute asthma attacks.

* Spinhaler is a registered trademark of Fisons plc.
† Rotahaler, Ventodisk, Becodisk and Diskhaler are registered trademarks of the Glaxo Group of Companies.
‡ Turbuhaler is a registered trademark of Astra Pharmaceuticals Ltd.

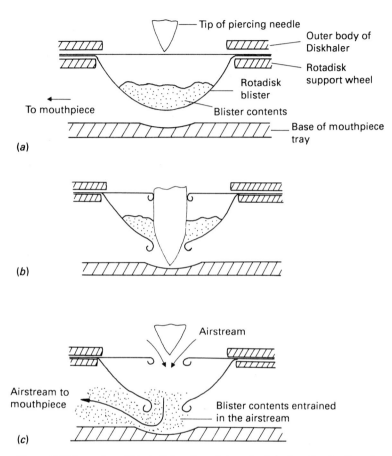

Figure 3.6 Dispersion of Ventodisk or Becodisk contents by breath actuation. A cross-section of Diskhaler is shown with a disc located on the support wheel. (*a*) A disc is located beneath an aperture in the body of the Diskhaler through which a piercing needle enters. (*b*) The needle penetrates the upper and lower surfaces of the blister. (*c*) The patient inhales through the device and pierced blister, entraining the blister contents into the airstream

Particle size analysis of therapeutic aerosols

As particle size is one of the major contributors to the efficacy of inhalation products, it has been necessary to develop appropriate techniques to examine the particle size and thus to estimate the respirable portion of inhalation aerosols. The *British*

Pharmaceutical Codex 1973 and *United States Pharmacopeia XX-NF (1980)* describe tests involving a microscopic evaluation of a slide on to which an aerosol emitted from a suspension-type pressure pack has impacted. The requirement is that the majority of the particles should be <5 µm in diameter, but this ignores the fact that the aerosol particles and droplets are constantly changing in size and velocity on inhalation by the patient.

Ideally, any sizing technique should be based on the principal mechanism pertinent to the dynamic aerosol fractionation within the respiratory tract, i.e. inertial impaction. Cascade impactors are devices of this nature, consisting of a series of jets, each followed at a precise distance by an impaction plate. Particles moving in an airstream collect on a plate placed in the path of the airstream, if their momentum overcomes the drag exerted by the airstream as it moves around the collection plate (Figure 3.7). Each jet is smaller than the preceding one, so that the velocity of the airstream and hence of the particles is

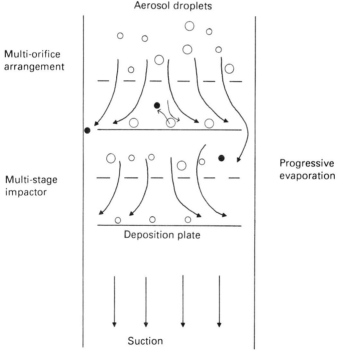

Figure 3.7 Diagrammatic representation of the theory underlying aerosol size analysis using a cascade impactor

increased as the aerosol cloud advances through the impactor. As a result, smaller particles eventually acquire sufficient momentum for impaction. In the characterization of therapeutic aerosols, it is common for a glass or metal tube with a smooth 90-degree bend to precede the first stage; the tube is designed in this way to mimic the constraints made on the inhaled aerosol cloud by the oropharynx.

Cascade impactors are subdivided into dry-stage and wet-stage devices, depending on whether the impacting particles deposit on a dry collection plate (normally stainless steel or glass), or on the surface of a pool of liquid. With dry-stage impactors, rebound of aerosol particles can occur, leading to re-entrainment of relatively large particles into the airstream and deposition on lower stages of the instrument. This will result in erroneous estimates of aerosol size distribution, but can be minimized by coating the plates with a viscous, silicone fluid to improve collection efficiency. A multistage liquid impinger (Figure 3.8) is a wet-stage device in which three of the four

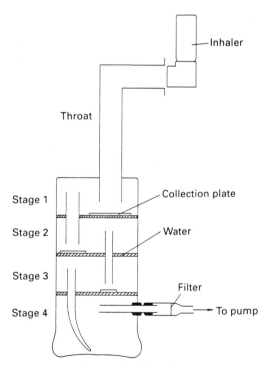

Figure 3.8 A multistage liquid impinger

stages comprise a wet sintered-glass collection plate and the fourth is a nozzle located tangentially to the surface of the collection solvent.

During the operation of these devices, air is drawn through the instrument at a precise velocity, usually by means of a vacuum pump located downstream of a filter placed after the final stage of the instrument. For evaluation of pressurized metered-dose inhalers, a predetermined number of actuations is fired into the airstream and the concentration of drug at each stage of the instrument is assayed chemically after each stage has been washed with a suitable solvent. Aerosols from nebulizers and powder inhalers can be characterized in a similar manner, although with the latter it is important to use an impactor which operates at a sufficiently high flow rate (>60 l/min) to empty the contents from the capsule.

Depending on the number of stages, complete aerosol characterization can be a tedious and time-consuming task, that may be acceptable during formulation development but is undesirable for routine quality assurance of manufactured products. A twin-stage device is recommended for such applications, where particles collected in the throat and stage 1 are considered to be non-respirable components of the aerosol cloud, and particles collected in stage 2 are equivalent to the respirable fraction. This has been designated an official test in the *British Pharmacopoeia 1988*, where a method is described for determination of the deposition of the emitted dose from pressurized inhalations using one of two twin-stage instruments. Modern techniques of sizing using laser instrumentation based on Doppler velocimetry or Fraunhofer diffraction have recently been applied to therapeutic aerosols. By coupling such instruments to computers with appropriate software, it is possible rapidly and easily to calculate size distributions of aerosol particles perturbing the laser beam. Ultimately these may replace inertial impaction as the method of choice for aerosol characterization.

References

1. Task Group on Lung Dynamics: deposition and retention models for internal dosimetry of the human respiratory tract. Report for International Commission on Radiological Protection. *Health Physics*, **12**, 173–207, 1966
2. Brain, J. D. and Valberg, P. A. Deposition of aerosols in the respiratory tract. *American Review of Respiratory Disease*, **120**, 1325–1373, 1979

3. Gonda, I. A semiempirical model of aerosol deposition in the human respiratory tract for mouth inhalation. *Journal of Pharmacy and Pharmacology*, **33**, 692–696, 1981
4. Stahlhofen, W., Gebhart, J. and Heyder, J. Biological variability of regional deposition of aerosol particles in the human respiratory tract. *American Industrial Hygiene Association Journal*, **42**, 348–352, 1981
5. Simonsson, B. G. Anatomical and pathophysiological considerations in aerosol therapy. *European Journal of Respiratory Diseases*, **63** (Suppl. 119), 7–14, 1982
6. Stout, S. A. and Derendorf, H. Local treatment of respiratory infections with antibiotics. *Drug Intelligence and Clinical Pharmacy*, **21**, 322–329, 1987
7. Hicks, R. Pulmonary fibrosis: allergies, dust diseases and drugs. *Pharmacy International*, **5**, 304–309, 1984
8. Ranney, D. F. Drug targeting to the lungs. *Biochemical Pharmacology*, **35**, 1063–1069, 1986
9. Bend, J. R., Serabjit-Singh, C. J. and Philpot, R. M. The pulmonary uptake, accumulation, and metabolism of xenobiotics. *Annual Review of Pharmacology and Toxicology*, **25**, 97–125, 1985
10. Clarke, S. W. and Newman, S. P. Therapeutic aerosols. 2. Drugs available by the inhaled route. *Thorax*, **39**, 1–7, 1984
11. Sturgess, J. M. Mucociliary clearance and mucus secretion in the lung. In *Toxicology of Inhaled Materials* (eds H. P. Witschi and J. D. Brain), Springer-Verlag, Berlin, pp. 319–367, 1985
12. Roth, R. A. and Wiersma, D. A. Role of the lung in total body clearance of circulating drugs. *Clinical Pharmacokinetics*, **4**, 355–367, 1979
13. Lourenço, R. V. and Cotromanes, E. Clinical aerosols. 1. Characterization of aerosols and their diagnostic uses. *Archives of Internal Medicine*, **142**, 2163–2172, 1982
14. Morén, F. Pressurized aerosols for oral inhalation. *International Journal of Pharmaceutics*, **8**, 1–10, 1981
15. Newman, S. P. and Clarke, S. W. Nebulisers: uses and abuses. *Archives of Disease in Childhood*, **61**, 424–425, 1986
16. Beasley, R., Rafferty, P. and Holgate, S. T. Adverse reactions to the non-drug constituents of nebuliser solutions. *British Journal of Clinical Pharmacology*, **25**, 283–287, 1988
17. Geddes, K. C. and Boyd, I. Microbial contamination of hospital nebulisers. *Pharmaceutical Journal*, **241** (Suppl: Practice Research), R23, 1988
18. Barnes, K. L., Clifford, R. and Holgate, S. T. Bacterial contamination of home nebulisers. *British Medical Journal*, **295**, 812, 1987
19. Editorial. Nebulisers and paradoxical bronchoconstriction. *Lancet*, ii, 202, 1988
20. Hughes, B. Practical nebulisation. *Chemist and Pharmacy Update*, 8–10, August 1989

Further reading

Benford, D. J. and Bridges, J. W. Xenobiotic metabolism in lung. In *Progress in Drug Metabolism, Vol. 9* (eds J. W. Bridges and L. F. Chasseaud), Taylor and Francis, London, pp. 53–94, 1986
Byron, P. R. Some future perspectives for unit dose inhalation aerosols. *Drug Development and Industrial Pharmacy*, **12**, 993–1015, 1986
Ganderton, D. and Jones, T. M. (eds) *Drug Delivery to the Respiratory Tract*, Ellis Horwood, Chichester, 1987

Morén, F., Newhouse, M. T. and Dolovich, M. B. (eds) *Aerosols in Medicine: Principles, Diagnosis and Therapy*, Elsevier, Amsterdam, 1985

Morrow, P. E. Factors affecting hygroscopic aerosol deposition in airways. *Physiological Reviews*, **66**, 330–376, 1986

Phalen, R. F. (ed) *Inhalation Studies: Foundations and Techniques*, CRC Press, Boca Raton, 1984

Walton, W. H. (ed), *Inhaled particles IV*, Parts 1 & 2, Pergamon Press, Oxford, 1977

Widdicombe, J. (ed) *Respiratory Pharmacology*, Pergamon Press, Oxford, 1981

4

Transdermal drug delivery

K. A. Walters

Introduction

For many years, attempts have been made to treat systemic disease by the application of medicaments to the skin. Several ancient cultures used ointments and plasters in the belief that they would alleviate a variety of symptoms. In some cases the formulations were active but this was more by chance than design. For example, the ancient Greeks used a mixture of water, olive oil and lead oxide as a balm. The efficacy of this formulation was probably attributable to the astringent properties of lead oxide and the emollient activity of the olive oil and this cannot, therefore, be considered as a transdermal delivery system because the effect was the result of activity of the formulation *on* the skin. For the purposes of this chapter a transdermal drug-delivery system is defined as a formulation that is applied to the skin and is designed to deliver the active drug across the skin, into the systemic circulation and subsequently to receptor sites remote from the area of application.

The use of the skin as a portal of entry to the systemic circulation was not significantly exploited until the 1950s. Before this time the skin was viewed as a physiological barrier that was not permeable enough to allow the passage of sufficient quantities of drugs to attain therapeutic blood levels. The development of ointments containing such agents as nitroglycerin (glyceryl trinitrate) and salicylates largely dispelled this notion, simply because they were shown to be therapeutically effective. Angina, for example, can be controlled for several hours by applying an ointment containing 2% nitroglycerin. Similarly, topical salicylates can be absorbed through the skin into arthritic joints. An overriding problem with these semisolid preparations, however, was (and still is) one of control. Drug concentrations in plasma and duration of action are not reliably predictable for several reasons, most of which are patient dependent. The dosage frequency, amount and area of application can affect therapeutic efficacy but the most significant factors are the inter- and intra-individual variation in skin permeability. The pioneering work of Scheuplein and Blank[1] opened a floodgate of research into skin penetration which finally resulted in the development of the controlled transdermal drug delivery systems available today.

This volume is concerned with alternatives to the oral route of drug delivery. Why alternatives to this widely used route are necessary has been fully discussed elsewhere, as have the specific advantages of transdermal therapy[2]. For completeness, however, the latter are briefly outlined here. Transdermal devices are easy to apply, can remain in place for up to 7 days (depending on the system), and are easily removed following or during therapy; patient compliance is thereby improved. The reduced dosing frequency and the production of controllable and sustained plasma levels tend to minimize the risk of undesirable side-effects sometimes observed after oral delivery (Figure 4.1). Although the viable epidermis contains enzyme systems capable of catabolizing many drugs[3], the avoidance of hepatic first-pass metabolism is an obvious advantage.

There are, of course, limitations to transdermal drug delivery, not least of which is the intrinsic barrier property of the skin. This is fully discussed in a later section; suffice it to say, for introductory purposes, that the physicochemical characteristics of the permeating molecule are the major determinants of the

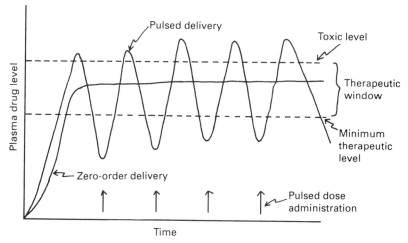

Figure 4.1 Drug concentration profiles in plasma following pulsed and zero-order delivery

rate and extent of transdermal absorption. Thus, at present, marketed transdermal delivery systems are available for only a few, highly potent drugs (scopolamine, nitroglycerin, oestradiol and clonidine), although several other candidates (for example, nicotine, timolol, testosterone, midazolam maleate) are at various stages of development.

Many of the drugs under investigation do not possess, intrinsically, any great ability to cross the skin and ways must be found to improve delivery. This could involve the use of prodrugs designed in such a way that they are more rapidly absorbed than the parent compound, yet are metabolized to the active species before receptor-site occupancy. Physical methods, such as iontophoresis, may aid the permeation of ionic drug species or the barrier may be chemically modified by the use of penetration enhancers. These developmental strategies should increase the number of candidate transdermal drugs in the near future. Another major obstacle limiting transdermal therapy is the possibility of allergic or irritant responses to the drug or other formulation constituents, the most obvious of which are the adhesives. At this time there is no way to predict, from a knowledge of the chemical structures involved, the probability of occurrence of this type of problem.

It is the purpose of this chapter to describe transdermal drug delivery systems and their use. An essential aspect of the understanding of these systems is a knowledge of the nature of the skin and its barrier properties. These are briefly discussed, together with factors affecting, and methods used to increase, skin permeability. This is followed by a discussion of the design, development and clinical usefulness of marketed transdermal systems. Finally, an attempt is made to predict the possible future of this route of drug delivery.

Skin structure and barrier properties

The barrier

The skin is a multilayered organ that is complex in both structure and function. Macroscopically, two distinct layers are apparent: the outer epidermis and the inner dermis (Figure 4.2). The dermis is composed of a network of collagen and elastin fibres embedded in a mucopolysaccharide matrix, which also contains blood vessels, lymphatics and nerve endings, thereby providing physiological support for the epidermis. Because the blood vessels approach the interface of the two layers very

81

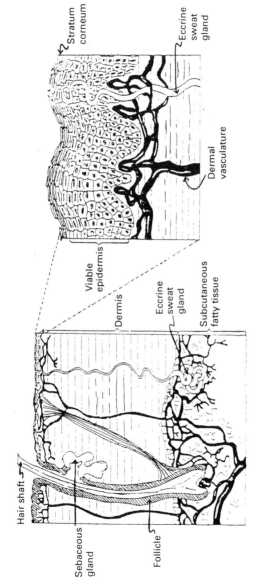

Figure 4.2 Schematic cross-section of the skin. Full-thickness skin is shown on the left and an expansion of the upper epidermal layers on the right. (Courtesy of Mr M. Walker)

closely, the dermis cannot be considered as a significant barrier to inward drug permeation *in vivo*. The epidermis comprises the viable epidermis and the stratum corneum. The viable epidermis comprises a layer of cells that undergo continuous differentiation to produce the stratum corneum, which is the outermost layer of skin. The viable epidermis is often regarded as having the properties of an aqueous gel and, as such, does not present a significant barrier to penetration in most circumstances. If the stratum corneum is damaged, or if extremely lipophilic drugs are being used, the viable epidermis can act as a rate-limiting factor in percutaneous absorption.

The stratum corneum is the major source of resistance to the penetration and permeation of the skin by drug molecules. This coherent membrane, which is 15–20 μm thick over much of the human body, consists primarily of blocks of cytoplasmic protein matrices (keratins) embedded in extracellular lipid. The keratin-containing cells (corneocytes) are arranged in an interlocking structure somewhat akin to bricks and mortar (Figure 4.3). In humans, the extracellular mortar consists of a structured

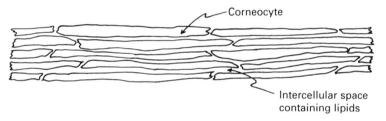

Figure 4.3 Schematic cross-section of the stratum corneum showing the interlocking arrangement of the corneocytes

complex containing several groups of lipids (Table 4.1). Identification of these lipids by solvent extraction and thin-layer chromatography has demonstrated a considerable degree of variability between body regions. Furthermore, the relative amounts of lipid groups apparently present can be significantly affected by the solvents used for extraction. It is generally agreed, however, that most of the human stratum corneum lipid consists of ceramides and neutral lipids such as free sterols, free fatty acids and triglycerides. The remainder is made up of phospholipids, glycosphingolipid and cholesterol sulphate, the last being of considerable importance to the desquamation process. Despite the very low levels of phospholipid, stratum corneum lipids are capable of forming bilayers, suggesting that

Table 4.1 Major lipids of the stratum corneum*

Lipid type	Amount (wt %)
Neutral lipids	64.6
Free sterols	14.0
Sterol esters	6.1
Free fatty acids	19.3
Triglycerides	25.2
Sphingolipids	18.1
Glycosphingolipids	2.6
Ceramides	15.5

* Abdominal region.

the intercellular space consists of lamellar liquid crystals (Figure 4.4). These broad sheets, which contain predominantly saturated lipids, comprise the major epidermal barrier to water and hydrophilic permeants[5].

The bricks are the dead, flattened cells of the horny layer, the corneocytes, which contain very little lipid. Their major structural components are aggregates of keratins arranged as bundles of individual keratin filaments. It has been recognized for many years that keratin is not a single substance but is a complex mixture of proteins, the most important chemical feature of which is the preponderance of the sulphur-containing diamino acid cystine[6]. The process of keratinization is complex and results in specific deposition of different keratins at various sites within and around the corneocyte. The thickened cell envelope, for example, consists of a protein–lipid–carbohydrate mixture in which the protein is rich in disulphide bonds. Most of the amorphous protein within the cell matrix is also rich in disulphide bonds, whereas the fibrous protein of the filaments does not appear to be so tightly cross-linked. Thus, the strength and durability of the stratum corneum is provided by the amorphous matrix protein surrounding the filaments and the membrane protein surrounding the cells.

The stratum corneum is breached by hair follicles and sweat ducts, which could, theoretically, provide a low-resistance rapid diffusion pathway across the skin. This shunt pathway may be significant for extremely slow penetrants, such as polar steroids, but the relatively small surface area of the follicles suggests that, for most penetrants, transepidermal permeation dominates except during the period immediately after application[7]. This concept is illustrated in Figure 4.5.

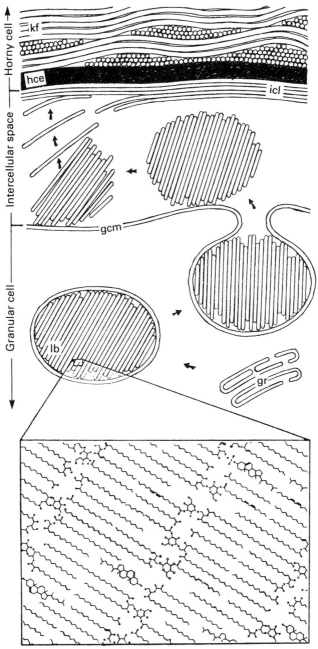

Figure 4.4 Representation of the formation of the stratum corneum. Lamellar bodies (lb), assembled in the Golgi region (gr) and endoplasmic reticulum within the epidermal granular cell membrane (gcm), are expelled into the intercellular space and rearrange into intercellular lamellae (icl) lying parallel to the corneocyte envelope (hce) and its keratin filaments (kf). Expanded insert shows the proposed arrangement of granular cell lipids into multiple bimolecular leaflets. (Adapted from reference 4)

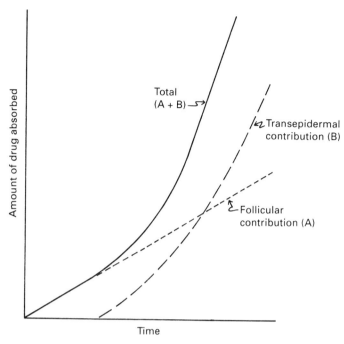

Figure 4.5 Contribution of diffusion through sweat ducts and hair follicles (A) and across the stratum corneum (B) to the early time course of skin penetration

Routes of penetration

It is clear that the structure of the stratum corneum offers two potential routes for drug permeation: one transcellular, the other via the tortuous but continuous intercellular lipid. The route through which permeation occurs is largely dependent on the physicochemical characteristics of the penetrant, the most important being the relative ability to partition into each skin phase. Each phase of the membrane can be characterized in terms of a diffusional resistance (R) which is usually defined in terms of the thickness (h) of the phase, the permeant diffusion coefficient (D) within the phase, and the partition coefficient (K) between the membrane phase and external phase such that:

$$R = \frac{h}{DK} \qquad (4.1)$$

or

$$P = \frac{DK}{h} \tag{4.2}$$

where P is defined as the permeability coefficient. The permeability coefficient is related to membrane flux (J) by:

$$J = AP\Delta C \tag{4.3}$$

in which ΔC is the difference in permeant concentration across the membrane, and A is the area of application. Combining Equations 4.2 and 4.3:

$$\frac{J}{A} = \frac{DK\Delta C}{h} \tag{4.4}$$

From Equation 4.4 it is evident that three major variables account for differences in the rate at which different drugs permeate the skin: the concentration of drug in the vehicle, the partition coefficient of the drug between the stratum corneum and the vehicle, and the diffusivity of the drug within the stratum corneum.

For a homologous series of chemicals, lipid/water partition coefficients increase exponentially with increasing alkyl chain length[8]. Thus, for a membrane of fixed or normalized thickness, the permeability coefficient through a lipid pathway will directly reflect partitioning tendencies and will follow:

$$P_n = P_{(n=10)}10^{\pi n} \tag{4.5}$$

In this equation, n is the alkyl chain length, $P_{(n=10)}$ is an intercept value equating to the homologue with no alkyl chain, and π is a positive constant related to the free energy of partitioning of a methylene unit. This relationship holds as long as the rate-determining step in crossing the membrane is passage through a lipid region; the equation indicates that, for a pure lipid membrane, a plot of the logarithm of the permeability coefficient versus the alkyl chain length of the permeant will be a straight line with an intercept at $P_{(n=10)}$ and a slope equal to π. Skin, however, is not a pure lipid membrane and a plot of the log of the permeability rate versus permeant lipophilicity appears sigmoidal, reflecting the existence of 'hydrophilic' pathways across the membrane (Figure 4.6). More polar homologues would permeate, preferentially, through these aqueous regions; there is, therefore, no partitioning dependency in the initial part of the curve. There is a further loss of direct partitioning sensitivity in the mass transfer process at

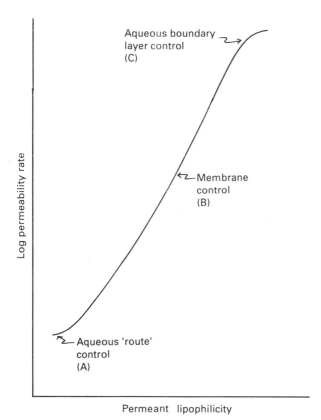

Figure 4.6 Plot of the log of the permeability rate versus permeant lipophilicity indicating the rate-controlling regions

higher permeant lipophilicity (Figure 4.6, region C); this is attributable to the emerging significance of a barrier of hydrophilic nature, known as the aqueous boundary layer. In skin this boundary layer is largely represented by the viable epidermis, a region of considerable hydrophilicity, which can present a significant resistance to the permeation of highly lipophilic compounds. This suggests, therefore, that drugs with partition coefficients indicating an ability to dissolve in both oil and water would be ideal candidates for transdermal delivery.

The mobility of a permeating molecule within a specific membrane phase can be numerically described by a diffusion coefficient. This parameter, represented by D in Equation 4.4, depends, to a large extent, on the degree of interaction between the diffusant and the surrounding medium, and tends to decrease with increase in permeant molecular volume (V):

$$D \propto V^{-1/3} \tag{4.6}$$

This relationship suggests that only a slight variation in diffusivity occurs with an increase in molecular size. However, any factor that tends to promote interaction between the permeant and the membrane will hinder diffusion. For example, the presence of extra hydroxy groups on the steroid oestriol results in a 45-fold decrease in diffusivity compared with oestrone [9].

There are a number of methods for determining membrane diffusivity, the simplest of which involves the generation of a permeation profile across the membrane *in vitro*. The data obtained from this type of experiment are usually expressed as a plot of cumulative amount of drug penetrated against time (Figure 4.7). The slope of the steady-state region gives the

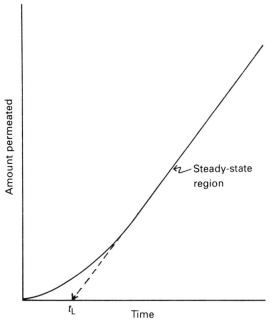

Figure 4.7 Plot of the amount of drug permeation as a function of time. Extrapolation of the steady-state region to the time axis indicates the lag time for diffusion (t_L)

permeant flux, or the amount of drug permeating through unit area of membrane in unit time. Extrapolation of the steady-state region to the time axis gives an intercept known as the 'lag time' (t_L), which is the time required for a permeant to establish a linear concentration gradient across the membrane, and represents the time of onset of maximal flux.

Provided that the thickness of the membrane is known, and that the membrane is homogeneous, the lag time provides an estimate of diffusivity. Thus, for a membrane of thickness h, the diffusivity D of a permeant with a lag time of t can be obtained from:

$$t = \frac{h}{6D} \tag{4.7}$$

Problems arise, however, in applying this simple lag time/ diffusivity relationship to biological membranes, such as the stratum corneum. There is no doubt that the average lipophilic diffusional path length in this case is greater than the membrane thickness. In addition, sorption or binding of the permeant to membrane components can increase lag time. Despite these drawbacks, the quantitation of lag times, which can vary from a few minutes to several days, is an important factor in the development of transdermal therapeutic systems. A full review of the mathematical approach to the early time course of absorption is given in an excellent analysis by Dugard[10].

Factors affecting skin absorption

For the most part, the previous section dealt with the influence of permeant physicochemical properties on skin transport properties. There are, however, several physiological factors that can affect the rate and extent of percutaneous absorption[11]. Perhaps the most significant to transdermal therapy is the hydration state of the stratum corneum. Design considerations for transdermal patch systems require a backing layer that is impervious to the drug and other formulation excipients. This usually renders the system occlusive, which can lead to increased skin hydration and an accumulation of water between the system and the skin. The latter increases the potential for sub-patch microbial growth and therefore the risk that this could lead to problems associated with biotransformation of the drug on the skin surface.

Hydration of the stratum corneum has been shown to enhance, retard, or have no effect on the skin penetration rates of a variety of compounds. In the majority of cases, however, hydration results in a decrease in skin barrier properties. This has been well demonstrated for many penetrants including esters of salicylic acid, corticosteroids, caffeine, and ibuprofen (Figure 4.8). There are, however, no firm theories on the mechanisms underlying the hydration-induced enhancement of skin permeability. The collective data indicate that the action is mediated by aqueous solvation of the polar regions of the glycosphingolipids and ceramides present in the intercellular spaces. This is supported by the observation that hydration effects are much less marked in the nail plate, a tissue containing considerably less lipid than the stratum corneum.

Further biological factors that may affect the rate and extent of percutaneous absorption include age, sex and race. The last two factors do not create any significant problems in the design and usefulness of transdermal therapeutic systems. There is, for example, no information to suggest that male skin differs from that of the female in permeability characteristics. Any slight

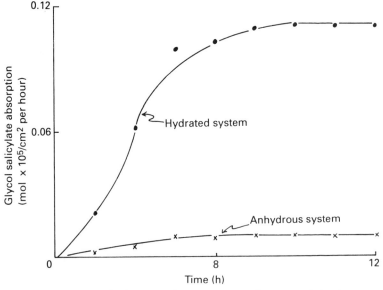

Figure 4.8 Influence of hydration on the percutaneous absorption of glycol salicylate, as determined by the urinary excretion of drug. (Adapted from reference 12)

differences that may occur are insignificant compared with variations among individuals. The data concerning differences between negroid and caucasian skin permeability indicate that black skin may be slightly less permeable that white skin, but no definite conclusions can be drawn because the available data are extremely limited.

For the most part, the intrinsic permeability characteristics of skin do not change with age: thus the rate of drug permeation across the skin of a full-term infant is much the same as that of an octogenarian. Blood concentration following the topical application of drugs, however, may be much higher in infants, whose surface-to-volume ratio is much higher than that of adults. Furthermore, although the existence of metabolic pathways within the skin is beyond doubt, the age at which significant levels of metabolic enzymes appear in the skin is unknown, nor is it known whether they diminish with age. Because the skin's permeability barrier does not start to develop until the last quarter of gestation, the skin of the premature infant is a less effective barrier than that of the full-term infant and this may lead to problems in fluid balance, temperature control and the application of medicaments to the defective barrier. The exploitation of the underdeveloped barrier in the premature neonate as a portal of entry for systemic drugs has been evaluated: the percutaneous application of theophylline was shown to be feasible [13].

One aspect of transdermal therapy that requires consideration at an early stage of the product development process concerns the site of application of the patch. The skin is not uniformly permeable over the entire body surface: several studies have demonstrated that the skin of the scrotum, palms, soles and postauricular area is much more permeable to drugs than skin from the back, chest, forearm or thigh (Figure 4.9). The properties of the stratum corneum vary at different body sites: the variations include differences in thickness, number of cell layers, stacking of cells, the amount of surface lipid and, perhaps most importantly, the relative amounts of different intercellular lipids.

Other factors that may influence site variation in per-cutaneous absorption include differences in the number and distribution of appendages and the depth of indentation of the dermal papillae into the epidermis, which may alter the temperature of the skin surface. Whatever the reason for the differences in skin permeability characteristics, they have been exploited in transdermal therapy. Thus, in the alleviation of

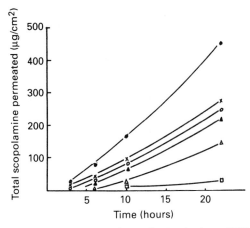

Figure 4.9 Permeation of scopolamine *in vitro* at 30°C through human skin from various sites: ●, postauricular; ×, back; ○, chest; ▲, stomach; △, forearm; □, thigh. (Adapted from reference 14)

motion sickness with transdermal scopolamine, the postauricular area is the preferred site of application. Another example is the preparation of transdermal testosterone for the treatment of hypogonadism, which is designed for application to the scrotum. There are, however, psychological, cosmetic and other reasons which limit the use of these relatively highly permeable areas. The postauricular area, for example, can accommodate only a small system such as the scopolamine patch. Larger transdermal systems are usually applied to the torso where they are not obvious and, in the case of transdermal glyceryl trinitrate, psychologically acceptable. Another important aspect regarding the site of application concerns the possibility of the patch causing irritation. In this case it is advisable to avoid repeated application to the same site and site rotation may be recommended; whereas this would be difficult to achieve at the postauricular or scrotal sites, the torso has a large enough surface area to accommodate this regimen.

Cutaneous metabolism

As outlined previously, the major barrier to the ingress of dermally applied chemicals is the stratum corneum. The nature of this membrane suggests that passive diffusion is the sole mechanism of transport. Immediately below this layer, however, are the cells of the viable epidermis which continually undergo differentiation and keratinization to replace the keratinocytes lost during the normal process of epithelial turnover. Although it is generally accepted that the viable epidermis is not a significant barrier to the diffusion of most chemicals, it is the most metabolically active layer in skin and is capable of chemically modifying a variety of permeating molecules. The metabolic processes catalysed by the enzymes present in skin include oxidation, reduction, hydrolysis and conjugation; the last process includes glucuronide and sulphate formation, methylation and glutathione conjugation.

Some of the enzyme systems present in skin can be illustrated by a consideration of steroid metabolism. For example, hydrocortisone is converted to cortisone under the influence of hydroxysteroid dehydrogenases. Similarly, oestradiol is oxidized to oestrone. The carbonyl groups of several steroids can be reduced to secondary alcohols. Thus, hydrocortisone, testosterone and progesterone are all potential substrates for cutaneous ketoreductase (Figure 4.10) or 5α-reductase (Figure 4.11). The majority of conjugation reactions with steroids involve sulphate conjugation, suggesting that the skin contains sulphokinase activity. A fuller description of the metabolic pathways within the epidermis can be found in the review by Noonan and Wester[3].

The presence of bacterial enzymes on the skin surface provides another potential inactivation pathway for topically applied drugs, one that would clearly be more significant in the environment beneath a transdermal patch. Attempts have been made to quantitate total cutaneous metabolism: for example, in the rhesus monkey, 15–20% of applied nitroglycerin is metabolized during the percutaneous absorption process[16]. Results from this type of study are often expressed as a skin/liver activity ratio (Table 4.2) which, for the viable epidermis, can vary from 80 to 240%.

The metabolic pathways encountered during percutaneous absorption may be used to advantage in the development of dosage forms containing prodrugs or 'soft' drugs. A prodrug is an inactive agent that is metabolized to the active, usually during the process of absorption and distribution. Prodrugs are designed in such a way that their physicochemical characteristics are more suited to the route of administration, which usually involves a modification of water/lipid solubility characteristics resulting in an alteration in partitioning tendencies. An example of this approach involves the use of the 1-butyryloxy-

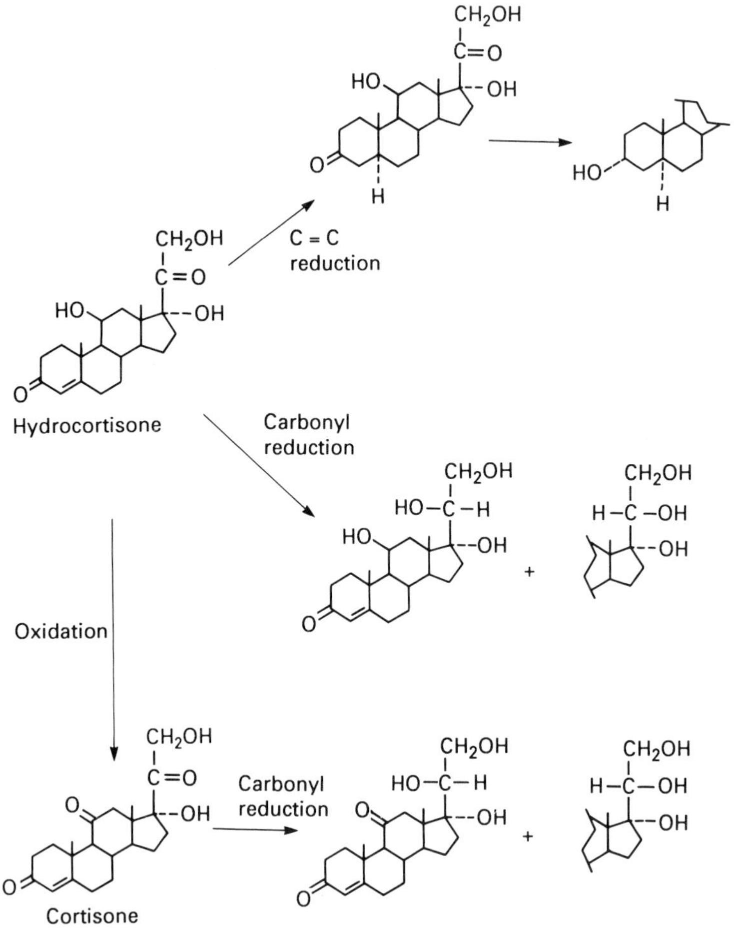

Figure 4.10 Various routes of skin metabolism for hydrocortisone. (Adapted from reference 15)

methyl derivative of 5-fluorouracil (Figure 4.12) which pene-trates the skin more effectively than the highly polar parent compound. Once the stratum corneum has been breached, the analogue is hydrolysed to generate the active drug. In general, the prodrug has no intrinsic pharmacological activity. On the other hand, soft drugs are defined as active compounds that are rapidly and predictably metabolized to inactive compounds once the therapeutic responses have occurred. For obvious

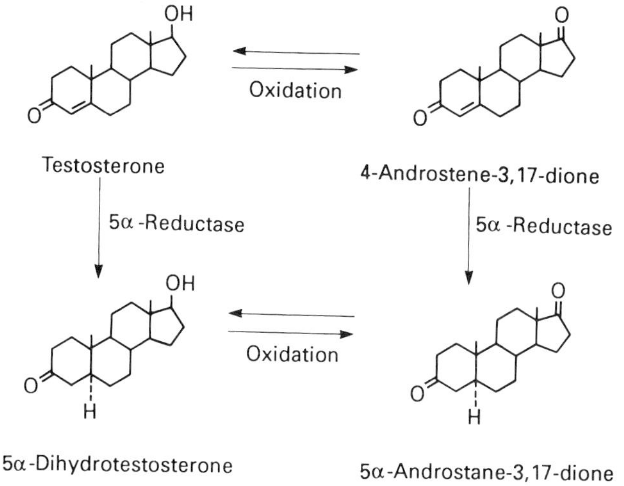

Figure 4.11 Routes of metabolism of testosterone in skin (Adapted from reference 15)

Table 4.2 Enzyme activity ratios in skin compared with liver

	Activity ratio (skin/liver)	
Enzyme/enzyme system	Whole skin	Epidermis
Aromatic hydrocarbon hydroxylase	0.02	0.80
7-ethoxycoumarin O-deethylase	0.02	0.80
Aniline hydroxylase	0.06	2.40
NADPH-cytochrome-c_2 reductase	0.06	2.40

Source: reference [3].

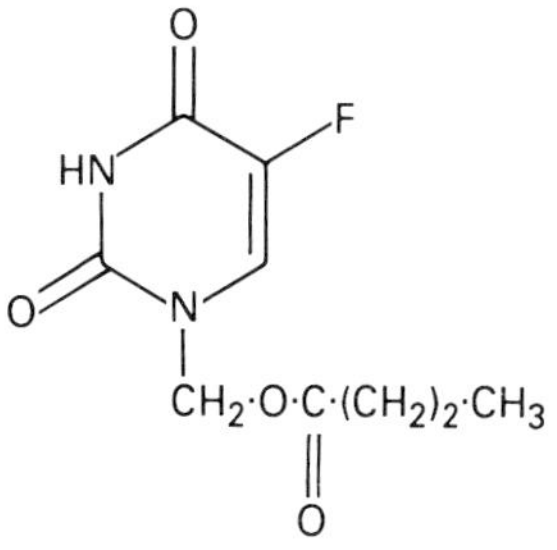

Figure 4.12 The 1-butyryloxymethyl derivative of 5-fluorouracil

reasons, this type of drug has limited usefulness in transdermal therapy but may prove highly desirable in the treatment of dermatological disorders.

Pharmacokinetics of transdermal absorption

The application of several simple mathematical relationships to the process of skin permeability has been discussed previously (pages 85–89). Although these models are useful for analysis of basic diffusion parameters, they have limited value in the prediction and determination of overall bioavailability profiles. In order to assess the feasibility of the transdermal route, several factors, including metabolism, rate of absorption and elimination, must be considered. This is, perhaps, best illustrated by the work of Guy and colleagues [17], who developed the kinetic model for topical drug delivery shown schematically in Figure 4.13. The various rate constants can be described as follows: $K(in)$ is dependent on the design of the transdermal patch and represents a release rate from the device; as is described in a later section (page 122), this release rate will be either first- or zero-order, with most patches demonstrating both characteristics. There may be the possibility of some back diffusion from the stratum corneum to the patch; this phenomenon, which is likely to be insignificant in most cases, is represented by the rate constant $K(r)$. $K(1)$ and $K(2)$ are the diffusion rates of the compound across the stratum corneum and viable epidermis, respectively. The reverse rate constant, $K(3)$, reflects partitioning such that $K(3)/K(2)$ is the stratum corneum/viable epidermis partition coefficient. It has been suggested that this partition coefficient can be predicted empirically from $K/5$,

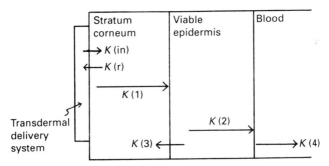

Figure 4.13 Linear kinetic model for percutaneous absorption. (Adapted from reference 17)

where K represents the octanol/water partition coefficient of the permeating molecule. $K(4)$ signifies the plasma clearance rate constant.

This model has been used to predict the plasma concentration of transdermally administered nitroglycerin and clonidine as a function of time. These profiles are shown in Figures 4.14 and 4.15, where they are compared with actual data from studies *in vivo*. Several other compounds, including oestradiol, scopolamine and timolol, also show remarkable similarities between predicted and actual plasma concentration profiles, suggesting that the model is useful for evaluating the feasibility of potential transdermal drug delivery candidates.

Although the model above provides predictive quantitative data based mainly on physicochemical parameters, other aspects of the percutaneous absorption process are more difficult to predict. Of most concern is the potential for metabolic degradation of the drug, either on, or during transit through, the skin. The major problem here is that only limited data are available on quantitative aspects of cutaneous metabolism. Modelling is possible, however, by estimating metabolic rate constants ($K(M)$) and varying the magnitude of

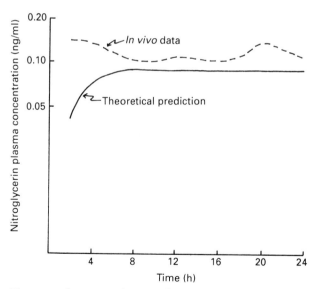

Figure 4.14 Comparison between theoretical prediction and plasma concentration *in vivo* versus time profile for nitroglycerin. (Adapted from reference 17)

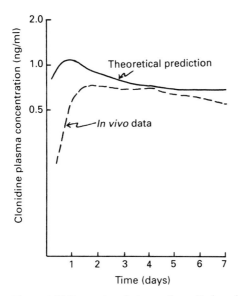

Figure 4.15 Comparison between theoretical prediction and plasma concentration *in vivo* versus time profile for clonidine. (Adapted from reference 17)

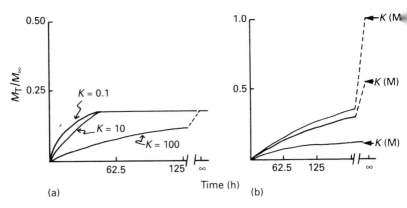

Figure 4.16 Effect of stratum corneum/viable epidermis partition coefficient (*K*) and epidermal metabolism kinetics (*K*(M)) on the fraction of the applied drug which reaches the cutaneous circulation. (*a*) Effect of varying *K* with a fixed *K*(M) of 0.1. (*b*) Effect of varying *K*(M) with a fixed *K* of 100. (Adapted from reference 17)

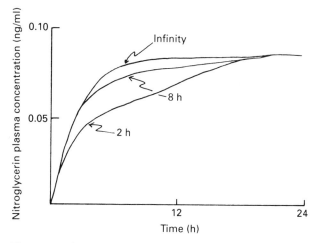

Figure 4.17 Effect of microbial degradation on the plasma concentration versus time profile following transdermal delivery from a membrane-moderated system containing a 2 mg priming dose. Half-lives for metabolism are indicated alongside the curves. (Adapted from reference 17)

$K(3)/K(2)$, which, effectively, alters the residence time of the drug in the skin. This results in profiles such as those shown in Figure 4.16. Profile (a) demonstrates the effect of varying $K(3)/K(2)$ with a fixed $K(M)$. Clearly, the more lipophilic drug ($K(3)/K(2) = 100$), having a relatively long residence time in the skin, will be more affected by cutaneous metabolic enzymes and be less bioavailable than its hydrophilic counterparts. A greater alteration of overall bioavailability can be predicted when the metabolic rate is varied with a constant $K(3)/K(2)$: in this case, profiles such as those shown in Figure 4.16b can be expected.

Estimation of the effects on bioavailability of surface metabolism by the skin's resident microflora can be made using half-lives for metabolism obtained *in vitro*. The plasma concentration profiles shown in Figure 4.17 illustrate the effects of varying metabolic half-lives from 2 h to infinity. Although the requisite plasma level is reached in all cases, the time taken to achieve that level is greatly extended as a result of metabolic activity. An obvious way to reduce this effect is to increase the amount of drug in the priming dose normally associated with the patch adhesive. However, as pointed out by Guy and colleagues[17], the lack of quantified cutaneous metabolic rate constants signifies that their simulations remain theoretical.

Skin-permeability enhancement

The ultimate success of any transdermal system depends on the ability of the drug to permeate skin in sufficient quantities to achieve therapeutic plasma levels. Unfortunately, many of the drugs under investigation do not possess, intrinsically, any great ability to cross the skin, and ways must be found to modify the diffusional barrier. This can be achieved chemically by the use of penetration enhancers, or physically by the use of such techniques as iontophoresis. Many of the chemical penetration enhancers are solvents or surfactants but several miscellaneous compounds do not fit easily into either category and will be discussed separately.

Solvents

In an earlier section (pages 89–90) the effect of hydration on skin-permeability properties was discussed. It appears that, in the majority of cases, stratum corneum hydration results in an increase in drug transport. Although most transdermal patch formulations contain little or no water, there is no doubt that the occlusive nature of many of these systems will result in hydration of the underlying skin. This can have significant implications, not only for the penetration rate of the therapeutic agent, but also on the occurrence of irritation and the possibility of sub-patch microbial growth. In these respects, water can be considered as a penetration enhancer, but it is unique in that it is inherent in skin.

Several other solvent groups can increase skin permeability. The lower alcohols, for example methanol and ethanol, have been found to be useful in this respect. The enhancing ability of these alcohols appears to be related to their capacity for extracting stratum corneum lipids and, in most cases, the increase in permeation rate is slight because only the polar lipids are significantly affected. The addition of a more hydrophobic cosolvent, such as n-hexane or n-dodecane, greatly enhances the activity of the alcohol. Other simple solvents capable of increasing penetration across skin include propylene glycol, acetone and tetrahydrofurfuryl alcohol. The latter two are of academic interest only, because toxicity considerations render it unlikely that they will ever be included in a product formulation.

The alkylmethyl sulphoxides, in particular dimethyl sulphoxide (DMSO) and decylmethyl sulphoxide ($C_{10}MSO$), are capable of markedly increasing skin permeability. Although the specific mode of action of DMSO is unresolved, it is likely that it involves extraction of stratum corneum lipids, lipoproteins and nucleoproteins, displacement of 'bound' water and delamination of the horny layer. This type of irreversible alteration of the stratum corneum is one reason curtailing the usefulness of DMSO in transdermal systems, but the major drawback is that significant permeability enhancement is obtained only when it is present at concentrations >70% (Figure 4.18). The C_{10} homologue, decyl methyl sulphoxide, has greater potential as an enhancer because it is effective at lower concentrations than DMSO. Indeed, C_{10}MSO has been approved by the FDA for use with tetracycline in the treatment of acne.

Several pyrrolidones have been examined to determine their ability to enhance penetration across skin. Most noteworthy are 2-pyrrolidone and N-methyl-2-pyrrolidone (Figure 4.19), both of which have shown penetration-enhancing activity for a diverse group of compounds including steroids, ibuprofen and aspirin. The primary site of action of the pyrrolidones appears to be on the polar route of penetration and this may be linked to their intrinsic humectant activity.

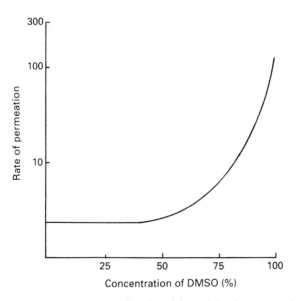

Figure 4.18 Permeation of methanol through hairless mouse skin in dimethylsulphoxide/water mixtures. (Adapted from reference 18)

Laurocapram (1-dodecylazacycloheptan-2-one; Azone) was the first compound specifically designed and synthesized as a skin penetration enhancer. A glance at the structure (Figure 4.19) reveals that it possesses many features of other more traditional enhancers. Early studies with Azone have shown it to be an effective enhancer for both hydrophilic and hydrophobic permeants. As with most penetration enhancers, the mode of action of Azone remains elusive but the indications are that it involves an alteration of the intercellular lipid regions of the stratum corneum.

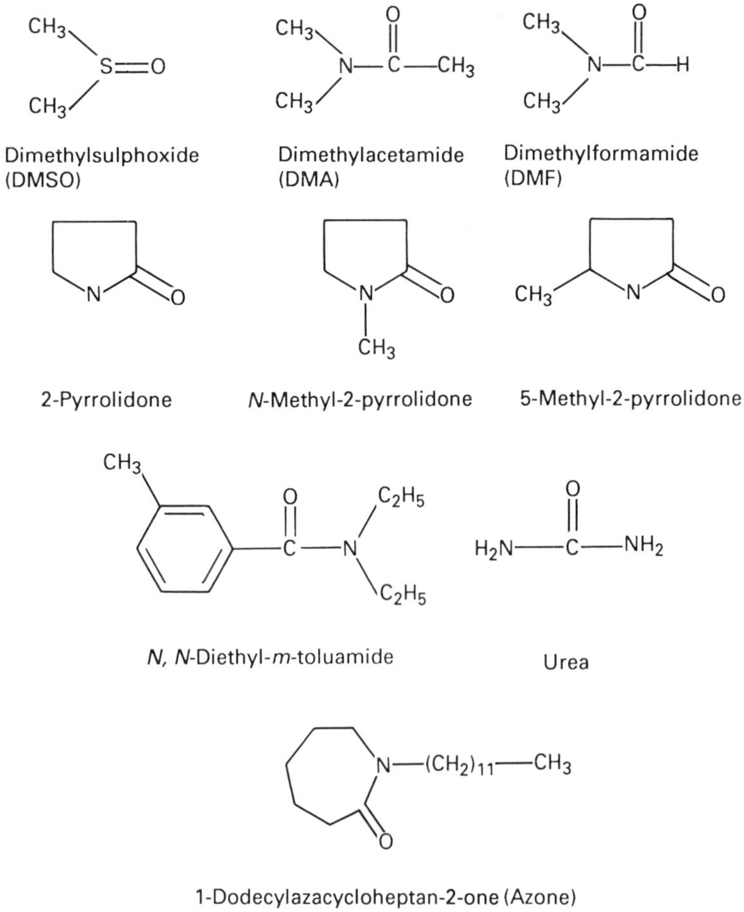

Dimethylsulphoxide (DMSO)

Dimethylacetamide (DMA)

Dimethylformamide (DMF)

2-Pyrrolidone

N-Methyl-2-pyrrolidone

5-Methyl-2-pyrrolidone

N, N-Diethyl-m-toluamide

Urea

1-Dodecylazacycloheptan-2-one (Azone)

Figure 4.19 Structures of several reported penetration enhancers

Surfactants

Surfactants are major components of pharmaceutical and cosmetic formulations. These substances are characterized by the presence of both polar and non-polar groups on the same molecule. In biological systems the effect of surfactants is complex, particularly their effect on cell membranes which can lead to alterations in permeability patterns. Increase in membrane transport at low surfactant concentrations can be attributed to the ability of the molecule to penetrate and eventually to disrupt the cell membrane structure. Reduction of transport of a permeant in surfactant systems is usually a result of surfactant micelle formation and is normally observed only if interaction between micelle and permeant occurs (Figure 4.20).

The classification of surfactants is based on the charge carried by the hydrophilic 'head' group. Thus, they can be anionic (e.g. sodium dodecyl sulphate), cationic (e.g. cetyltrimethyl ammonium bromide) or non-ionic, in which case the polar group is

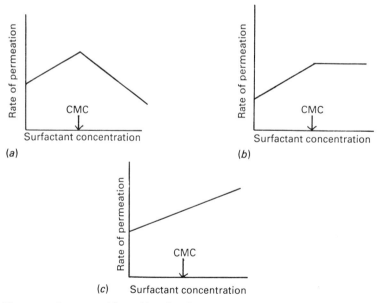

Figure 4.20 Some possible profiles of surfactant-induced alterations in membrane penetration. (a) Enhancement followed by a strong permeant/micelle interaction; (b) enhancement followed by a moderate permeant/micelle interaction; (c) enhancement with no permeant/micelle interaction. The arrow denotes the surfactant critical micelle concentration (CMC)

normally a polyoxyethylene chain (e.g. polyoxyethylene sorbitan monopalmitate). Occasionally, a further classification is necessary because the surfactant has the ability to behave either as a cation or anion, depending on the pH of the solution; these compounds are ampholytic and can also exist in a non-ionic form (e.g. N-dodecyl-N,N-dimethyl betaine). The hydrophobic portion of surfactants usually consists of flexible alkyl or aryl chains.

Anionic surfactants can penetrate and interact strongly with skin, the amount penetrating being dependent on surfactant structure, principally on the alkyl chain length. The most widely studied surfactants in this group are the alkyl sulphates, which can penetrate and destroy the integrity of the stratum corneum within hours following application. For example, sodium dodecyl sulphate can significantly enhance the permeation of several diverse chemicals including water, chloramphenicol, naproxen and naloxone. As with their intrinsic permeability, the degree of barrier alteration induced by these surfactants is dependent on the alkyl chain length, the dodecyl and tetradecyl moieties being the most effective. The action of these surfactants on skin is undoubtedly related to their ability to interact with, and bind to, epidermal proteins.

Although significant increases in skin penetration can be achieved using anionic surfactants it is unlikely that they will find a use in transdermal therapeutic systems, primarily because of their irritation potential.

Cationic surfactants are reputedly more irritant than the anionics and they have not, therefore, been widely studied as skin-penetration enhancers. Despite this, they have been shown to enhance the permeation of several chemicals.

The fact that many of these long-chain alkyl amines are protonated at the slightly acidic pH of the skin surface, yet become deprotonated at neutral pH, has stimulated investigations into the possibility of facilitating the transport of ionized drugs across skin (Figure 4.21). At the outer skin surface the amine has the capacity to form an ion pair with the drug. The ion pair then diffuses down its own concentration gradient to the inner layers of the stratum corneum. In this region (pH 7.4) the amine deprotonates, liberating the anion, and is then free to travel back to the skin surface. Only small amounts of amine are required for the carrier mechanism, which has been shown to function in artificial membranes. There are also indications that it can function in skin: for example, the skin-penetration rate of salicylate can be enhanced by several related amines, including

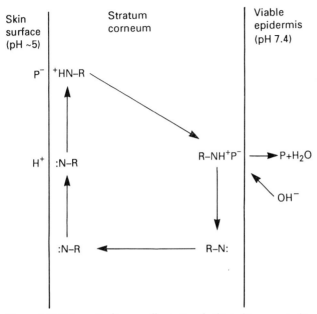

Figure 4.21 Schematic diagram illustrating facilitated transport of ionizable drugs using a carrier mechanism: N–R, long-chain substituted amine; P, drug. (Adapted from reference 19)

oleylamine (a primary amine with a mono-unsaturated C18 alkyl chain), polyoxyethylene-5-oleylamine and bis-(2-hydroxyethyl) cocoamine, the latter being the most effective. It is difficult to determine any definite structure–activity relationship for the alkyl amines but it is apparent that increasing the degree of ethoxylation reduces the efficiency of these compounds to act as skin-penetration enhancers. With the primary amines, as with most surfactant species, the dodecyl analogue appears to be a more effective enhancer than those with a longer alkyl chain.

Of the three major classes of surface-active agents, non-ionics have long been recognized as those with the least potential for irritancy. Although there are many different types of non-ionic surfactants, the majority of studies concerning their effects on biological systems are limited to four principal series: these are the polysorbates, polyethoxylated alkyl ethers and esters, polyethoxylated alkyl phenols, and poloxamers (which are polyoxyethylene–polyoxypropylene 'ABA' block co-polymers). Polysorbates 20, 40, 60 and 80 increase the flux of several drugs across skin, and when applied in conjunction with propylene glycol the surfactants are more effective enhancers. There is little doubt that monomers of this group can interact with skin and alter its barrier properties. The micelles, however, have a marked solubilizing capacity which, for interacting molecules, can lead to a significant decrease in permeant thermodynamic activity in the vehicle and thereby can reduce penetration rates.

Polyoxyethylene alkyl ethers and esters have been shown to enhance the percutaneous absorption of naloxone, griseofulvin, proquazone, diflorasone diacetate, flufenamic acid, nicotinic acid and methyl nicotinate. For surfactants of the polyoxyethylene alkyl ether type, the magnitude of penetration enhancement depends on the length of both the alkyl and the polyoxyethylene chain; surfactants with an alkyl chain length of C12 linked to an ethylene oxide chain of 10–14 units have been found to be the most effective (Table 4.3). In most cases the surfactant-induced enhancement of penetration is greatest for more polar permeants (Figure 4.22).

Polyoxyethylene aryl ethers have been widely used as solubilizing agents for membrane-bound enzymes. The limited data available on the effects of this type of surfactant on skin permeability characteristics, however, suggest that their enhancer potential is minimal. Similarly, the poloxamers appear to be minimally effective as skin-penetration enhancers unless they are used in combination with other enhancers such as DMSO.

The collective data for non-ionic surfactants suggest that their mode of action on the skin is related to their ability to partition

Table 4.3 Influence of surfactant chain length on the enhancement of skin permeation of methyl nicotinate

Alkyl chain length	Ethylene oxide chain length	Increase in permeation (%)
8	10	5
12	10	99
16	10	67
18	10	70
16	2	13
16	6	66
16	14	55
16	20	15
16	30	12
16	45	12
16	60	39

Data from reference [20].

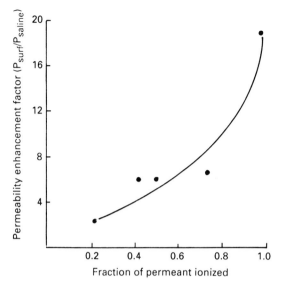

Figure 4.22 Enhancement of the skin permeation of nicotinic acid using a non-ionic surfactant; effect of varying the degree of ionization of the permeant. (Data from reference 21)

into the intercellular lipid phases of the stratum corneum. This results in increased fluidity in this region, which presumably reduces diffusional resistances. The lack of skin-permeability-enhancing activity for those surfactants with branched chains or aromatic groups in their hydrophobic portions suggests that these compounds are not as readily incorporated into the lipid structure of the stratum corneum. It is likely that, at high surfactant concentrations, some lipid extraction will occur, further reducing diffusional resistance.

Another possible mode of action involves penetration of the surfactants into the intracellular matrix followed by interaction and binding with the keratin filaments. This mechanism appears optimal for dodecyl-based surfactants. It is possible that both mechanisms discussed above are operative to some degree.

Long-chain fatty acids have been shown to be effective penetration enhancers for a variety of drugs, provided that they are applied in a suitable cosolvent such as propylene glycol. This is also true for the corresponding alcohols. The presence of *cis*-double bonds in the alkyl chain appears to increase the degree of enhancement over the corresponding saturated acid

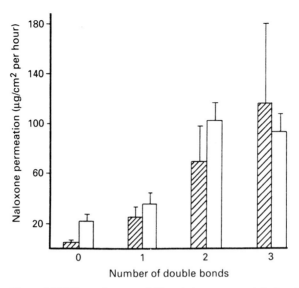

Figure 4.23 Effects of saturated (0) and *cis*-unsaturated (1, 2 and 3) fatty acids and fatty alcohols on the penetration of naloxone across skin. Alkyl chain length C18; ☐ , fatty acids; ▨ , fatty alcohols. (Adapted from reference 22)

or alcohol (Figure 4.23). The degree of penetration enhancement is dependent on several factors including chain length, position, type (*cis* or *trans*) and number of double bonds[23].

Miscellaneous chemicals

Urea (Figure 4.19) has been shown to enhance the permeation of several compounds across skin, the most notable being hydrocortisone. It is present in several marketed dermatological formulations including moisturizers and steroid creams. Urea is capable of increasing hydration of the stratum corneum and also has keratolytic effects. It has recently been proposed that urea may lower the phase transition temperature of stratum corneum, causing increased fluidity at ambient temperature[24]. Because of the proteolytic effects of urea, however, its safety in long-term usage is questionable.

Calcium thioglycolate has been widely used as a depilatory and has been applied to the skin in concentrations ≤10%. The mechanism of action of this compound probably involves a disruption of the keratin matrix. The available evidence suggests that calcium thioglycolate can enhance the skin penetration of theophylline and 6-carboxyfluorescein without any appreciable damage. In view of its keratolytic properties, however, further toxicological evaluation is necessary.

Some potential penetration enhancers have recently been described but the available data on their effectiveness are sparse. These include eucalyptol, di-*O*-methyl-β-cyclodextrin and soybean casein.

Physical methods for enhancing skin penetration

In the previous sections, enhancement of skin penetration by the use of chemicals has been described. In addition to these 'traditional' methods of reducing the barrier function of skin some physical methods have also been demonstrated: the two most often cited are iontophoresis[25] and phonophoresis[26].

Iontophoresis

Iontophoresis involves the migration of charged molecules under the influence of an electrical current. The basic premise assumes that an ionized drug can be driven across the skin by placing an electrode of similar charge to the drug in the donor system and the electrode of opposite charge either under the skin or at a surface area remote to that of drug application (Figure 4.24). The transdermal delivery of several drugs has been shown to be enhanced by iontophoresis: these include

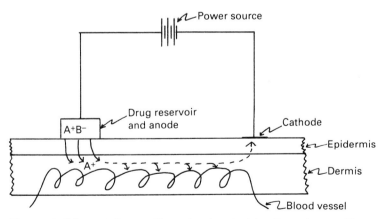

Figure 4.24 Schematic diagram illustrating the principle of iontophoresis. The drug (A^+) permeates across the epidermis and migrates towards the cathode. During this process the drug is available to the cutaneous microcirculation

local anaesthetics (e.g. lignocaine), β-blockers (e.g. metoprolol, propranolol) and insulin. The latter is generating considerable interest in view of the lack of alternative routes for the delivery of the macromolecule to diabetic patients. Although research into the feasibility of a transdermal iontophoretic insulin delivery device is still in the early stages, there is good reason for optimism. Glycaemic control can be achieved rapidly (Figure 4.25) and maintained for several hours. There are, however, several problems to be addressed, not least of which are the development of a convenient portable device capable of producing different drug fluxes as required, evaluation of the immunogenic aspects of the transdermal delivery of insulin and determination of the optimum electrical parameters[28].

Although much progress has been made since the early (c. 1910) experiments, where patients were 'wired up' to mains

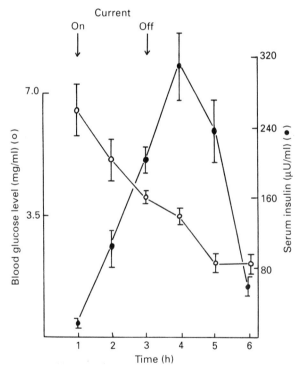

Figure 4.25 Influence of iontophoresis on the skin penetration of insulin using alloxan-diabetic rabbits. A current of 0.4 mA was applied for 2 h. (Adapted from reference 27)

electricity, there are still some disadvantages to be overcome in the field of transdermal iontophoresis. For example, burns are often produced by low voltage and can be caused without the sensation of pain. Additionally, electric shocks can be caused by a high current density at the skin surface. It may be possible to reduce these problems by applying a pulsed current, allowing the skin to recover during the 'current off' period. Despite the fact that the therapeutic applications of iontophoresis are not based on sound clinical data, several commercial systems are available[25].

Phonophoresis

Phonophoresis (sonophoresis) refers to the use of ultrasound to enhance the skin permeability of topically applied therapeutic agents[26]. This method has been used for >30 years as an adjunct to the topical treatment of skin disorders; as such it has been used in conjunction with steroids and antibiotics. More recently, phonophoresis has been used for the local transdermal delivery of macromolecules such as interferon and α-chymotrypsin.

   Although the mechanisms of action of ultrasound on stratum corneum permeability are not yet fully understood, there does appear to be a relationship between frequency level and depth of penetration in that lower frequencies have a greater ability to penetrate into the deeper layers of the skin. Whatever the mechanism of action, it does appear to be reversible and, provided that the correct frequency, power level and duration can be determined, phonophoresis may prove to be a safe technique for enhancing skin permeation in man.

Development of therapeutic systems

As with all pharmaceutical products, specific guidelines are established for the development of transdermal dosage forms. These guidelines encompass the use of GLP (Good Laboratory Practice) and GMP (Good Manufacturing Practice). Transdermal systems, however, are relatively new dosage forms and, at present, there are no specific regulatory demands. In the United Kingdom, transdermal therapeutic systems are regarded as medicinal products and need to follow the same regulatory procedures as more conventional preparations. It is not the intention here to discuss fully drug development programmes;

instead, this chapter concentrates on those aspects specific to transdermal delivery systems.

Design considerations

All transdermal delivery systems developed to date can be described on the basis of three design principles: drug in adhesive, drug in matrix (usually polymeric) and drug in reservoir (Figure 4.26). In the last the reservoir is separated from the skin by a rate-controlling membrane. When selecting a

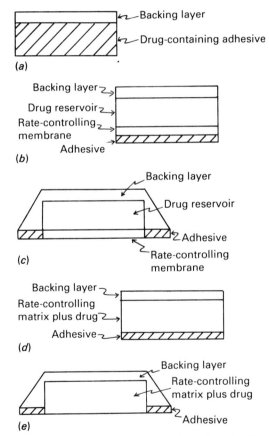

Figure 4.26 Cross-sections of some transdermal delivery systems. (a) Drug-in-adhesive matrix system; (b) membrane-controlled system; (c) membrane-controlled system with annular adhesive; (d) polymer matrix control system; (e) polymer matrix control system with annular adhesive

particular system, three critical considerations are necessary: adhesion to skin, compatibility with skin and the physical/ chemical stability of the total formulation and components.

All devices are secured to the skin by means of a pressure-sensitive adhesive. These adhesives, usually based on silicones, acrylates or polyisobutylene, can be evaluated by wear-testing and assessment of rheological parameters. Standard rheological tests include creep compliance (which will measure the ability of the adhesive to flow into surface irregularities), elastic index (which determines the extent of stretch or deformation as a function of load and time) and recovery following deformation. Skin-adhesion performance is based on several properties such as initial and long-term adhesion, lift and residue. The adhesive must be soft enough to ensure initial adhesion, yet have sufficient cohesive strength to remove cleanly, leaving no residue. Because premature lift will interfere with drug delivery, the cohesive and adhesive properties must be carefully balanced and maintained over the period of intended application. This can be evaluated only by wear-testing, in which a placebo patch is applied to skin.

Skin adhesion is affected by shape, conformability and occlusivity. Round patches tend to be more secure than those of sharply angled geometry. If the patch is able to conform to the contours of the skin it will resist lifting and buckling with movement. The presence of water may affect adhesive properties and therefore the occlusivity of the system must be taken into consideration. Occlusion for prolonged periods can lead to excessive hydration and the problems associated with microbial growth; this may increase the possibility of irritation or sensitization to the various components of the system. It is not unknown in pharmaceutical development for individual ingredients to be toxicologically inert but the assembled dosage form, optimized for drug-delivery requirements, to exhibit adverse toxicological characteristics. For transdermal delivery systems, safety evaluations must include not only the adhesive and drug but also backings, liners, membranes and reservoir components. Both acute and chronic toxicity tests should be performed, with special emphasis on the potential of the system to produce irritation and sensitization in long-term usage.

Although there are many differences in the design of transdermal devices, features are common to all systems: these include the liner, pressure-sensitive adhesive, backing layer and primary pack, all of which must, of necessity, be compatible for a successful device. For example, if a system is designed in such a way that the drug is intimately mixed with adhesive, or diffuses from a reservoir through the adhesive, the potential for interaction between drug and adhesive, which can lead to either a reduction of adhesive effectiveness or formation of a new chemical species, must be fully assessed. Similarly, the presence of residual monomers, catalysts, plasticizers and resins may react to give new chemical species. Additionally, it is possible that the excipients and/or their reaction products may interfere with adhesive systems. In order to determine potential incompatibilities within the system, differential scanning calorimetry coupled with elevated-temperature accelerated-storage tests should be conducted. Incompatibilities between the adhesive system and other formulation excipients, although undesirable, are not necessarily impeding: designs such as that shown in Figure 4.26c, in which the adhesive is remote from the body of the system, may be utilized.

A variety of materials can be used to fabricate the backing material and release liner (Table 4.4). The principal property of these materials is that they should be impervious to the drug and other formulation excipients. The most useful backing materials are those which conform with the skin and provide sufficient resistance to transepidermal water loss to allow some hydration of the stratum corneum, yet are able to maintain a healthy sub-patch environment.

Table 4.4 Examples of materials used in transdermal delivery devices

Backing materials	*Rate-controlling membranes*
Polyvinylchloride	Ethylene-vinyl acetate
Polyethylene (HD, LD)	Polypropylene
Polypropylene	Polycarbonates
Ethylene-vinyl acetate	Polyvinylchloride
Aluminium foil	Silicones
Polyesters	Cellulose acetate/nitrate
Non-woven rayon	
Nylon	*Reservoirs*
	Mineral oil
Release liners	Carboxypolymethylene
Polyethylene-coated paper	Polyacrylamide
Polyester fluoropolymer	Celluloses
Pressure-sensitive adhesives	*Polymer matrix reservoirs*
Silicones	Silicone elastomers
Rubbers	Rayons
Acrylates	Polyurethanes

The release liner must be easily separated from the rest without lifting off any of the pressure-sensitive adhesive to which it is bound. The liners are usually films or coated papers. Silicone release coatings are used with acrylate and rubber-based adhesive systems, while fluorocarbon coatings are used with silicone adhesives[29].

Drug incorporation

There are three principal methods for incorporating the active species into a transdermal system and this has led to the loose classification of patches as membrane, matrix or drug-in-adhesive types. It is, however, quite possible to combine the main types of patch, for example by placing a membrane over a matrix or using a drug-in-adhesive in combination with a membrane/matrix device in order to deliver an initial bolus dose.

The membrane patch uses a delivery rate-controlling membrane between the drug reservoir and the skin. Either microporous membranes, which act to control drug flux by the size and tortuosity of pores in the membrane, or dense polymeric membranes, through which the drug permeates by dissolution and diffusion, are used. Several materials can be used for such membranes, examples being ethylene vinyl acetate copolymers, silicones, high-density (HD) polyethylene, polyester elastomers and polyacrylonitrile. In general, the membrane should be permeable only to the drug and should retain other formulation excipients, unless skin-penetration enhancers are to be used in the delivery system, in which case the membrane should also be permeable to the enhancer. Another essential characteristic of the membrane is that it must be capable of delivering a constant amount of drug over the period of product application.

A variety of materials can be used for the drug reservoir: these range from simple formulations such as mineral oil, to complex formulations such as aqueous/alcoholic gels. The overriding requirement for the reservoir is that it must be capable of permitting zero-order release of the drug over the entire dispensing lifetime of the system. Essentially, this requires the reservoir material to be saturated with the drug over the period of product application, and this can be achieved by formulating the drug as a suspension. Examples of products marketed in this form include Transiderm-Nitro and Transderm Scop (Ciba-Geigy).

The second type of transdermal system is the matrix system, in which the drug is uniformly dispersed in a polymeric matrix through which it diffuses to the surface of the skin. The theory of dissolution and diffusion in polymeric matrices is complex and often difficult to model[30]. Several steps are involved in this process, principally dissociation of drug molecules from the crystal lattice, solubilization of the drug in the polymer matrix and diffusion of drug molecules through the matrix. Many variables may affect the rate of dissolution and diffusion of the drug, making it particularly difficult to predict release rates from experimental or prototype formulations. It is obvious, however, that for a drug to be released from a polymeric matrix under zero-order kinetics the drug must be maintained at an (ideally) saturated concentration in the fluid phase of the matrix and that the diffusion rate of the drug within the matrix must be much greater than the diffusion rate in the skin.

Several methods can be used to alter the release rate of a drug from a polymeric matrix. Some of these are illustrated by a recent study on the release of several drugs from silicone matrices[31]. Silicone medical-grade elastomers (polydimethyl-siloxanes) are flexible, lipophilic polymers with excellent compatibility with biological tissues. These polymers can be co-formulated with hydrophilic excipients, such as glycerol, and inert fillers, such as titanium dioxide, in order to alter release kinetics. Increasing the amount of glycerol in the matrix has been shown to increase the release rate of indomethacin, propranolol, testosterone and progesterone (Figure 4.27). The presence of the inert fillers, titanium dioxide or barium sulphate, tends to reduce the release rate. These data demonstrate the relative ease with which release rates of drugs can be altered to achieve a desired profile.

Other polymers that have been used as drug reservoirs in matrix-type systems include polyurethanes, polyvinyl alcohol and polyvinylpyrrolidones.

A variation of the matrix-type transdermal drug-delivery system is the microsealed delivery device. In this system the drug is dispersed in a reservoir which is then immobilized as discrete droplets in a cross-linked polymeric matrix (Figure 4.28). Release can be further controlled using a polymeric microporous membrane, and thus the system combines the principles of the reservoir and matrix-type devices. The rate of release of a drug from the microsealed delivery system is dependent on the partition coefficient between the reservoir droplets and the polymeric matrix, on the diffusivity of the drug

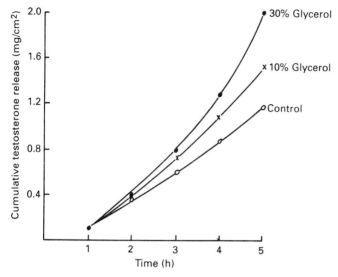

Figure 4.27 Enhanced release of testosterone from silicone matrices using glycerol. (Adapted from reference 31)

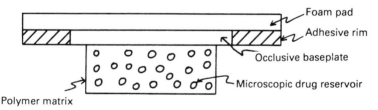

Figure 4.28 Cross-section of microsealed drug delivery device. See text for details

in the reservoir, the matrix and the controlling membrane, and on the solubility of the drug in the various phases. The combination of these factors results in zero-order release and there are, obviously, many ways of achieving a desired release rate. An example of a microsealed transdermal delivery device is Nitrodisc (Searle), which has been shown to be capable of maintaining a constant blood level of nitroglycerin during application (Figure 4.29).

Perhaps the simplest form of transdermal drug-delivery device is the drug-in-adhesive system, e.g. Nitro-Dur II (Key). This approach involves mixing the drug in an adhesive solution

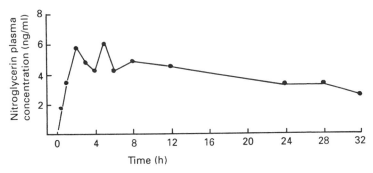

Figure 4.29 Plasma concentration versus time curve for nitroglycerin following application of microsealed transdermal system. (Adapted from reference 32)

which is then coated on to, for example, a polyester film to produce an adhesive tape. This simplicity is, however, deceptive. Several factors need to be considered, all of which are dependent on potential interaction between the drug and the adhesive. This can involve chemical interactions resulting in possible interference with adhesive performance, breakdown of the active species or formation of new chemical entities. Additionally, the physicochemical characteristics of the drug and adhesive system may result in different release rates for hydrophilic and hydrophobic drugs: for example, silicone adhesives are typically lipophilic, which limits the solubility of hydrophilic drugs within the adhesive matrix.

This type of problem is now being addressed by the major manufacturers of skin-compatible adhesives. As an example, the Dow Corning Corporation are evaluating the potential of a hydrophobic/hydrophilic silicone/organic copolymer which consists of polyoxyethylene oligomers grafted on to a siloxane backbone. By formulating these graft copolymers with silicate resins, a range of pressure-sensitive adhesives is obtained. Obviously, as the polyoxyethylene chain length is increased the adhesive becomes more hydrophilic, resulting in more rapid release of hydrophilic drugs. This does, however, reduce the optimum adhesiveness of the system, but acceptable adhesive properties can be obtained by reducing the molecular weight of the silicone resin. Clearly, much work remains to be done in the area of pressure-sensitive skin-compatible adhesives, but the outlook is promising.

Biopharmaceutical considerations

A fundamental consideration in the development of transdermal therapeutic systems is whether the dermal delivery route will provide the requisite bioavailability for drug effectiveness. This is determined by the skin-penetration rate of the drug, the potential for drug metabolism during diffusion across the skin and the biological half-life of the drug.

Penetration rate can be predicted from the physicochemical properties of the drug and may be modified, if necessary, by the use of penetration enhancers. Drug metabolism and plasma clearance, however, cannot be influenced by any simple means. Although the prediction of skin penetration and bioavailability of drugs from transdermal therapeutic systems using the model shown in Figure 4.13 has been shown to be remarkably accurate [2], there is no doubt that testing of formulated patches *in vitro* and *in vivo* will continue as the most accurate means of evaluating their potential usefulness. Unfortunately, a wide variety of experimental approaches have been developed and it is only recently that guidelines have been laid down in an attempt to rationalize this aspect of pharmaceutical development [33]. The best way to determine bioavailability in man is to measure penetration in human subjects by analysing plasma levels of drugs following application. These data can then be compared with the corresponding data following parenteral delivery.

In the earlier stages of product development, skin penetration rates from prototype patches are usually determined *in vitro* using diffusion cells of a variety of designs (Figure 4.30), and skin from a variety of animals. Obviously, the system *in vitro* will provide little information on the metabolism and distribution of the drug following absorption, but a major advantage is that experimental conditions can be controlled precisely in such a way that the only variables are in the prototype. In the latter stages of product development, human skin should be the membrane of choice in systems *in vitro*. It is doubtful that experimentation *in vitro* will ever eliminate the necessity of measurements *in vivo* but its value as a tool in the development process is without question.

From the above discussion it is apparent that an accurate determination of the pharmacokinetic profile of a transdermal delivery system is possible using both theoretical and practical methods. These will provide data on skin-penetration rates, plasma concentrations of drugs and their clearance, but will not

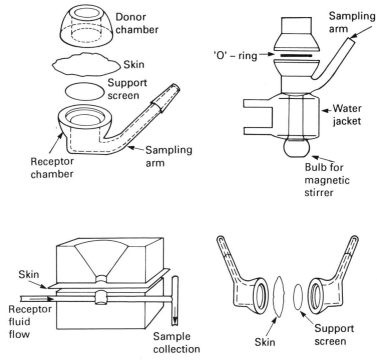

Figure 4.30 Examples of diffusion-cell designs for skin penetration studies *in vitro*. (Courtesy of Dr R. C. Scott)

provide answers to questions relating to pharmacodynamics. Is, for example, the attainment of a target steady-state drug plasma level any guarantee of therapeutic efficacy? Are all candidate drugs for transdermal delivery pharmacologically suitable for continuous administration? These questions remain to be answered but must be addressed when considering new molecules for transdermal delivery systems.

System manufacture and quality control

For the most part, the manufacturing processes for reservoir, matrix and drug-in-adhesive transdermal systems are similar, in that they involve the following stages: preparing the drug; mixing the drug (with penetration enhancer, if required) with the reservoir, matrix or adhesive; casting into films and drying (or moulding and curing); laminating with other structural components (e.g. backing layer, rate-controlling membrane and release liner); die-cutting and, finally, packaging (Figure 4.31). Casting and lamination are the most critical steps in the manufacturing process: tensions and pressures must be carefully controlled to provide a wrinkle-free laminate that ensures reproducible adhesive-coating thickness and uniform drug content.

As with all controlled-release delivery systems, final product checks include content uniformity, release-rate determination

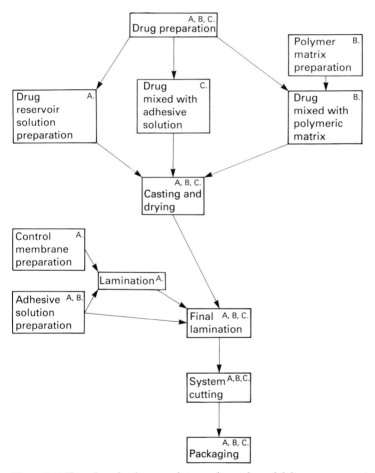

Figure 4.31 Flow chart for the manufacture of transdermal delivery systems. A, Membrane control systems; B, polymer matrix control systems; C, drug-in-adhesive matrix systems

and physical testing. The content-uniformity evaluation involves removing a random sample of patches from a batch and assaying the amount of drug present. At present there are no specific pharmacopoeial standards, but it has been recommended that the Capsule Content Uniformity requirements of the *United States Pharmacopeia (USP) XXI* be used as the general requirements for transdermal drug-delivery systems[34].

Of the several methods available for determining drug release rates from controlled-release formulations, the US PMA Committee[34] has recommended three: the 'Paddle Over Disk' (which is identical to the USP paddle dissolution apparatus except that the transdermal system is attached to a disk or cell resting at the bottom of the vessel that contains medium at 32°C); the 'Cylinder-Modified USP Basket' (which is similar to the USP basket method except that the system is attached to the surface of a hollow cylinder immersed in medium at 32°C), and the 'Reciprocating Disk' (in which patches attached to holders are oscillated in small volumes of medium, allowing the apparatus to be useful for systems delivering low concentrations of drug).

Much remains to be established in the field of pharmacopoeial standards for transdermal drug delivery systems. The various companies currently marketing these systems are applying their own rigorous quality control procedures, which are totally adequate, but standardized methodology is essential to the pharmaceutical industry.

Marketed transdermal systems

In the United States four drugs currently are approved for administration via the transdermal route: these are nitroglycerin, oestradiol, clonidine and scopolamine. Several other compounds, including nicotine, fentanyl, testosterone and timolol, are in various stages of the regulatory approval process.

Nitroglycerin

Nitroglycerin is a potent vasodilator that is used in the treatment of angina pectoris. The clinical utilization of nitroglycerin dates back over a century: oral and sublingual nitrates have been available for decades (page 30). By the early 1970s oral nitrate therapy for angina pectoris was thought to be of limited usefulness, mainly because of the rapid and almost total first-pass metabolism of the drug. The development of more sensitive assays, however, demonstrated that therapeutic plasma nitrate concentrations could be achieved after oral doses of nitroglycerin. Sublingual nitroglycerin formulations are the most efficient products for the treatment of acute angina attacks[35]. The effects of nitroglycerin following sublingual application are, however, short-lived and, in the search for an effective long-lasting therapeutic system, the skin was considered as an alternative route to the systemic circulation.

Transdermal administration of nitroglycerin was first evaluated in the 1950s using ointment formulations. As with any semi-solid preparation, however, it is virtually impossible to standardize the surface area and thickness of the applied layer and this results in irregular absorption and fluctuating plasma concentrations. None the less, these simple ointment formulations can provide effective anti-anginal therapy for periods of up to 8 h, which is considerably longer than the relief provided by sublingual administration. Plasma concentrations of nitroglycerin following the application of a 2% ointment are shown in Figure 4.32.

Attempts to attain predictable skin absorption of nitroglycerin led to the independent development of three transdermal delivery systems: Transiderm-Nitro (Ciba-Geigy), Nitro-Dur (Key) and Nitrodisc (Searle). These have been followed by

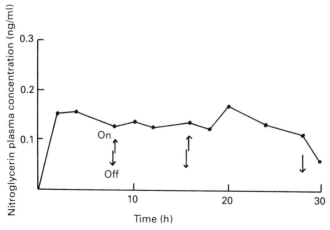

Figure 4.32 Plasma concentration versus time profile for nitroglycerin following application (arrows) of a 2% ointment formulation. (Adapted from reference 36)

several other systems incuding Deponit-TTS (Schwartz) and Nitro-Dur II (Key).

Transiderm-Nitro is a membrane-moderated system, whereas Nitro-Dur and Nitrodisc are based on the polymeric matrix type of device, the latter being a microsealed drug-delivery system. In these systems the nitroglycerin is normally incorporated as a lactose triturate. In the Nitro-Dur system, for example, nitroglycerin is distributed homogeneously throughout a polymeric matrix containing polyvinylpyrrolidone and poly(vinyl) alcohol. The system releases nitroglycerin linearly with the square root of time and, for a 10 cm^2 patch containing 51 mg, 80–90% of the drug is released over 24 h. The newer system, Nitro-Dur II, is a drug-in-adhesive device that contains nitroglycerin in acrylic-based polymer adhesives with a resinous cross-linking agent. This simple, but effective, system is available in a range of dosage strengths that are capable of delivering 2.5–15 mg in 24 h. All the systems described are capable of maintaining remarkably similar and constant plasma nitroglycerin concentrations over a 24 h period (Figure 4.33).

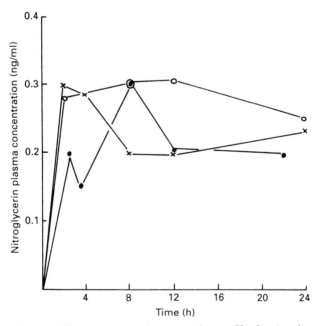

Figure 4.33 Plasma concentration versus time profiles for nitroglycerin following application of three different transdermal systems: ○, Nitrodisc; ×, Transiderm-Nitro; ●, Nitro-Dur. (Adapted from reference 2)

A potential disadvantage of the continuous transdermal delivery of nitroglycerin concerns the question of tolerance: it is apparent that a constant plasma level of the drug may compromise its pharmacological effect. There are two major types of tolerance, pharmacokinetic and physiological. The former is the result of increases in the rate of drug elimination with time, but it is unlikely that this is the cause of nitrate tolerance. Physiological tolerance is an adaptive process resulting from a loss of tissue responsivity (despite the maintenance of constant drug plasma concentrations) and is the most likely reason for nitrate tolerance. Recently, however, a major multicentre clinical trial involving three of the US-approved transdermal systems has been carried out. The evidence suggests that insertion of a 'nitrate-free' interval into the therapeutic regimen may counteract tolerance. The timing of this interval will depend on individual patients and whether anginal attacks are exercise-induced or nocturnal. Development of 'on-off' patches is currently under way, the idea being that the patch will be worn for 24 h but nitrate will not be delivered for the whole period. There is little doubt that the market for transdermal nitroglycerin is large enough to support the development of these more complex systems.

Oestradiol

The postmenopausal syndrome is characterized by a variety of symptoms including hot flushes, atrophic vaginitis, sleep disturbance and alterations of secondary sex characteristics. Many of these symptoms are the result of an imbalance in hormone levels due to a loss of endogenous oestrogen production. The more serious consequences of oestrogen deficiency are associated with the development of osteoporosis and atherosclerosis. Oral oestrogen replacement therapy, introduced in the 1960s, can relieve postmenopausal vasomotor symptoms, prevent osteoporosis and minimize atrophic changes in the vagina, but its use is associated with undesirable effects mainly related to elevated hepatic proteins (such as renin substrate) and non-physiological levels of oestrone[37]. These undesirable effects can be reduced by avoiding first-pass metabolism (as shown by their absence following parenteral delivery of oestradiol), suggesting that the transdermal route may prove advantageous.

As with the nitrates, a semi-solid formulation of oestradiol (Oestrogel, Besins Iscovesco) is available in Europe. This hydro-alcoholic gel has the disadvantage that methods of dosing are imprecise and plasma concentrations of oestradiol are large and variable.

Estraderm TTS (Ciba-Geigy) is a membrane-controlled transdermal system containing 17β-oestradiol. It has been demonstrated that the transdermal delivery of oestradiol is efficacious at a very low delivery rate of 0.025–0.1 mg/day, and twice-weekly application of the patch appears sufficient to maintain levels of oestrogen adequate for replacement. The serum levels of oestrogen following the transdermal application of three systems are shown in Figure 4.34. These systems, which differ in oestrogen content and surface area, show a good correlation between delivery surface area and serum concentration of drug [38].

A potential disadvantage of transdermal oestrogen is the possible increased risk of endometrial cancer resulting from continuous oestrogen administration. This risk can be reduced by the concomitant administration of progestogens. For this reason Estraderm TTS, which was introduced in the UK in 1987, is indicated only for hysterectomized women. A combined oestradiol/norethisterone acetate patch is currently in the latter stages of development.

For women sensitive to the adhesive in transdermal patches or intolerant to oral lactose, subdermal implants of plain oestradiol are a suitable alternative in hormone replacement therapy.

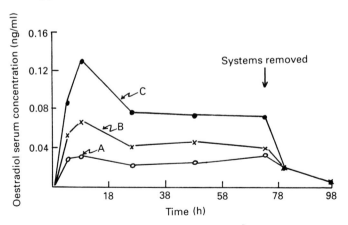

Figure 4.34 Serum concentration versus time profile for oestradiol following single applications of 5 cm² (A), 10 cm² (B) and 20 cm² (C) transdermal delivery systems. (Adapted from reference 38)

Scopolamine

Scopolamine is an extremely effective drug in the treatment of motion sickness. It is, however, frequently associated with side-effects such as drowsiness, sedation, blurred vision, cycloplegia and dry mouth. These effects are related to the parasympathomimetic properties of the drug following oral delivery, and can be reduced by administering scopolamine in a continuous low-dose regimen (Figure 4.35). This drug is therefore a prime candidate for rate-controlled transdermal delivery and, indeed, was the first compound to be successfully developed as a transdermal therapeutic system.

The Transderm-Scop device developed by Alza is membrane controlled, the membrane being a microporous polypropylene film. The drug reservoir is a solution of scopolamine in a mixture of mineral oil and polyisobutylene. Following an initial burst of drug, release from the reservoir is zero-order and is maintained over a 3-day period. The device is worn behind the ear, because skin permeability in this region is relatively good and ensures that the rate of drug release from the system determines the rate of entry into the circulation. The efficiency of the scopolamine transdermal system has been thoroughly tested under extreme conditions and there is little doubt that antiemetic levels of the drug are achieved and maintained. The system has been approved in the UK as Scopoderm TTS (Ciba-Geigy), and the three-day patch is marketed in numerous countries world wide. Currently, Ciba-Geiby are developing a once-daily patch.

Clonidine

Clonidine is a centrally acting antihypertensive agent that has been used effectively (alone or in combination with other drugs) for the oral treatment of mild, moderate or severe hypertension. The mechanism of action involves stimulation of α-adreno-ceptors in the brain stem, resulting in reduced sympathetic outflow from the central nervous system and decreases in peripheral vascular resistance, heart rate and blood pressure. Unfortunately, the use of clonidine is associated with side-effects such as drowsiness and dry mouth. Alza have developed a membrane-type transdermal therapeutic system containing clonidine that delivers the drug to the skin surface at a constant rate for at least 7 days; the pressure-sensitive adhesive contains a loading dose. Therapeutic plasma levels of clonidine are of the

128

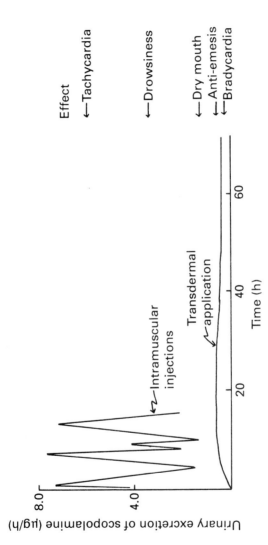

Figure 4.35 Comparison of urinary excretion of scopolamine following intramuscular injection and during transdermal administration. (Adapted from reference 39)

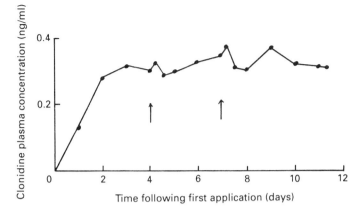

Figure 4.36 Plasma concentration versus time profile for clonidine following multiple applications of a transdermal system. Systems were applied at 0, 4, and 7 days. (Adapted from reference 40)

order of 0.6–1.2 ng/ml, requiring hourly release rates from the transdermal system of 1.5–2.0 μg/cm². Therapeutic plasma levels are attained 3–7 days after application, the long lag time being a function of the biological half-life of clonidine and a possible 'reservoir effect' for clonidine in the stratum corneum [2].

Plasma levels of clonidine following multiple applications of transdermal systems are shown in Figure 4.36. Recently, oral clonidine has been proposed as an aid to stopping smoking; the potential of using transdermal clonidine for this indication is, as yet, unresolved.

When clonidine was first introduced in a transdermal form there were a number of reports of skin reactions: indeed, 15–20% of patients treated showed local cutaneous reactions, including irritation and sensitization typical of contact dermatitis. Although in the majority of cases the reactions were mild, there have been reports of severe reactions (including erythema and vesiculation) after, on average, 20 weeks of transdermal therapy. For the most part, however, the mild reactions can be tolerated if the patient is instructed to change the application site at intervals of 3–5 days. This apart, the application of clonidine transdermally is well tolerated in most patients and is a beneficial addition to the antihypertensive armoury.

Products in development

In addition to the commercially available systems described above, several transdermal systems are in the later stages of development; these systems include devices for delivering nicotine, fentanyl, timolol, mepindolol and testosterone.

It is possible to produce significant systemic levels of nicotine by topical application. This has prompted the development of transdermal systems for nicotine which may be useful for those who wish to stop smoking. Certainly, the delivery of nicotine by this route would reduce the intake of the carcinogens present in smoke particulates, as well as intake of dangerous volatiles such as hydrogen cyanide and carbon monoxide. Transdermal nicotine would also have several advantages over other routes of administration: for example, direct contact of nicotine with the buccal mucosa, as occurs with nicotine chewing gum, often produces adverse effects such as heartburn and nausea. At least three pharmaceutical companies (Elan, Merrell Dow in conjunction with Alza, and Ciba-Geigy) are currently developing transdermal nicotine systems.

The transdermal delivery of narcotic analgesics has been practised haphazardly for several years. For instance, a small sponge soaked in morphine solution would be attached with an adhesive plaster to the skin of patients with terminal cancer, thereby providing continuous pain relief. A greater control over the amount of drug delivered can be achieved using a transdermal patch and, to this end, Alza and Janssen have jointly developed a transdermal fentanyl formulation. Fentanyl was originally developed by Janssen and has been marketed since 1968 as an intravenous formulation. The Alza patch provides controlled release of the drug for 72 h. In addition, Cygnus (an American specialist transdermal product development company) has independently developed a technique for delivering fentanyl through the skin, and the product is undergoing clinical trials.

Timolol and mepindolol are β-adrenoceptor-blocking agents which are very useful in the treatment of hypertension. Small-scale clinical trials of a transdermal patch system for mepindolol (developed by Pharmed and Smith Kline & French) suggest that reduction of blood pressure is significant after a week of therapy, with further improvements following 3 weeks of therapy. Timolol has also been found to be effective in reducing blood pressure following dermal application [41]. In this case the drug was applied in a semi-solid vehicle to the

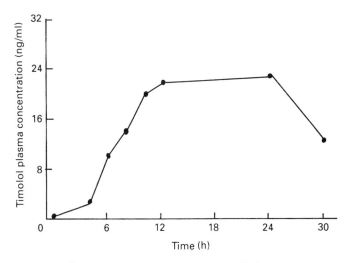

Figure 4.37 Plasma concentration versus time profile for timolol following application of 60 mg in a topical gel. (Adapted from reference 41)

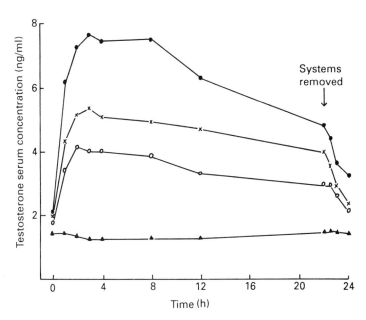

Figure 4.38 Serum concentration versus time profiles for testosterone following scrotal application of transdermal systems containing varying amounts of drug: ●, 15 mg; ×, 10 mg; ○, 5 mg; ▲, control. (Adapted from reference 42)

chest of six volunteers for 30 h; the resulting blood profiles (Figure 4.37) were sufficient to reduce systolic blood pressure and post-exercise heart rate.

Alza have developed a transdermal therapeutic system for the controlled delivery of testosterone. When this system was applied daily over 12 weeks to hypogonadal patients, serum testosterone levels were raised to the normal range. The delivery system is a self-adhesive testosterone-impregnated patch which is applied to the scrotum. When membranes containing 5, 10 and 15 mg testosterone are applied, the time course of serum testosterone concentration is dose dependent, as shown in Figure 4.38. Clearly, this system offers a viable and preferable alternative to the current means of treating testosterone deficiency, which is the intramuscular injection of a long-acting testosterone ester.

Concluding remarks

Transdermal drug delivery can be an extremely useful method for administering drugs. Unfortunately, the skin is designed to maintain a stable environment within the body and, to this end, has limited permeability to most molecules; at present, therefore drug delivery by this route is confined to very potent species. There are, however, ways to increase the rate of permeation through skin and specific examples were cited earlier. Although a number of penetration enhancers are known, so far only ethanol has appeared in a marketed product, but it is likely that Azone will soon achieve regulatory approval. Bearing in mind the amount of research being pursued in the area of skin-permeability enhancement, it is likely that these methods will form part of transdermal development, thereby increasing the number of drug candidates potentially available. If enhancers are included in a formulation, however, consideration must be given to the potential hazards of increasing the skin penetration rate not only of the drug but also of other formulation excipients – including the enhancer itself – which could lead to an increased incidence of irritation and other adverse responses.

Peptides and polypeptides are often quoted as being the drugs of the future and it is possible that sufficient amounts of these highly potent moieties could be delivered transdermally – provided that a safe and effective method for reducing the skin barrier can be found. Significant advances are being made, for example, in the transdermal delivery of insulin using ion-tophoresis. Once again, however, care must be exercised in the use of iontophoresis: recent evidence[43] indicates that the process can enhance the permeability rate of non-electrolytes, such as the alkanols. This raises two major questions: what is the mechanism underlying the effect of iontophoresis on the permeation of neutral molecules, and what are the implications with regard to the permeation of formulation excipients? Although the former is most likely to be attributable to a current-induced alteration in water movement, the latter question remains to be resolved.

As with all dosage forms, both advantages and disadvantages are associated with transdermal delivery systems. Good patient compliance, reduction of dosage frequency, reduction of side-effects, avoidance of first-pass metabolism and the produc-tion of sustained and controllable levels of drug in plasma, are probably the most significant advantages. The disadvantages include the inherent impermeability of skin, the elicitation of either allergic or irritant responses, and the possibility of biotransformation of the drug on its passage across the skin. Another potential problem is that the site of application may influence the plasma levels of drug. This difficulty is less significant if the patient is fully instructed on the positioning of the device. Overall, the advantages of transdermal drug delivery far outweigh the disadvantages.

This chapter provides a brief overview of the field of transdermal drug delivery. Although much remains to be done there are clear indications that systemic therapy via transdermal therapeutic systems will continue to gain greater prominence with the development of newer, more refined, systems.

References

1. Scheuplein, R. J. and Blank, I. H. Permeability of the skin. *Physiological Reviews*, **51**, 702–747, 1971
2. Guy, R. H. and Hadgraft, J. Transdermal drug delivery: a perspective. *Journal of Controlled Release*, **4**, 237–251, 1987
3. Noonan, P. K. and Wester, R. C. Cutaneous metabolism of xenobiotics. In *Percutaneous Absorption: Mechanisms, Methodology, Drug Delivery*, (eds R. L. Bronaugh and H. I. Maibach), Marcel Dekker, New York, pp. 65–86, 1985
4. Wertz, P. W. and Downing, D. T. Glycolipids in mammalian epidermis: structure and function in the water barrier. *Science*, **217**, 1261–1262, 1982
5. Madison, K. C., Swartzendruber, D. C., Wertz, P. W. and Downing, D. T. Presence of intact intercellular lipid lamellae in the upper layers of the stratum corneum. *Journal of Investigative Dermatology*, **88**, 714–718, 1987

6. Fraser, R. D. B., MacRae, T. P. and Rogers, G. E. *Keratins: Their Composition, Structure and Biosynthesis.* C. C. Thomas, Springfield, 1972
7. Scheuplein, R. J. Mechanisms of percutaneous absorption. II. Transient diffusion and the relative importance of various routes of skin penetration. *Journal of Investigative Dermatology*, **48**, 79–88, 1967
8. Flynn, G. L. and Yalkowsky, S. H. Correlation and prediction of mass transport across membranes. I. Influence of alkyl chain length on flux-determining properties of barrier and diffusant. *Journal of Pharmaceutical Sciences*, **61**, 838–852, 1972
9. Scheuplein, R. J., Blank, I. H., Brauner, G. J. and MacFarlane, D. J. Percutaneous absorption of steroids. *Journal of Investigative Dermatology*, **52**, 63–70, 1969
10. Dugard, P. H. Skin permeability theory in relation to measurements of percutaneous absorption in toxicology. In *Dermatotoxicology*, 3rd edn (eds F. N. Marzulli and H. I. Maibach), Hemisphere, Washington, pp. 95–120, 1987
11. Kligman, A. M. A biological brief on percutaneous absorption. *Drug Development and Industrial Pharmacy*, **9**, 521–560, 1983
12. Wurster, D. E. and Kramer, S. F. Investigations of some factors influencing percutaneous absorption. *Journal of Pharmaceutical Sciences*, **50**, 288–293, 1961
13. Evans, N. J., Rutter, N., Hadgraft, J. and Parr, G. Percutaneous administration of theophylline in the preterm infant. *Journal of Pediatrics*, **107**, 307–311, 1985
14. Shaw, J. E. and Mitchell, C. Dermal drug delivery systems. A review. *Journal of Toxicology, Cutaneous and Ocular Toxicology*, **2**, 249–266, 1984
15. Pannatier, A., Jenner, P., Testa, B. and Etter, J. C. The skin as a drug metabolizing organ. *Drug Metabolism Reviews*, **8**, 319–343, 1978
16. Wester, R. C., Noonan, P. K., Smeach, S. and Kosobud, L. Pharmacokinetics and bioavailability of intravenous and topical nitroglycerin in the rhesus monkey. Estimate of percutaneous first-pass metabolism. *Journal of Pharmaceutical Sciences*, **72**, 745–748, 1983
17. Guy, R. H., Hadgraft, J. and Bucks, D. A. W. Transdermal drug delivery and cutaneous metabolism. *Xenobiotica*, **17**, 325–343, 1987
18. Kurihara-Bergstrom, T., Flynn, G. L. and Higuchi, W. I. Physicochemical study of percutaneous absorption enhancement by dimethylsulfoxide: kinetic and thermodynamic determinants of dimethylsulfoxide mediated mass transfer of alkanols. *Journal of Pharmaceutical Sciences*, **75**, 479–486, 1986
19. Barker, N. and Hadgraft, J. Facilitated percutaneous absorption: a model system. *International Journal of Pharmacuetics*, **8**, 193–202, 1981
20. Walters, K. A., Walker, M. and Olejnik, O. Non-ionic surfactant effects on hairless mouse skin permeability characteristics. *Journal of Pharmacy and Pharmacology*, **40**, 525–529, 1988
21. Walters, K. A., Olejnik, O. and Harris, S. Influence of nonionic surfactant on the permeation of ionized molecules through hairless mouse skin. *Journal of Pharmacy and Pharmacology*, **36** (Suppl.), 78P, 1984
22. Aungst, B. J., Rogers, N. J. and Shefter, E. Enhancement of naloxone penetration through human skin in vitro using fatty acids, fatty alcohols, surfactants, sulfoxides and amides. *International Journal of Pharmaceutics*, **33**, 225–234, 1986
23. Cooper, E. R. Increased skin permeability for lipophilic molecules. *Journal of Pharmaceutical Sciences*, **73**, 1153–1156, 1984
24. Beastall, J., Guy, R. H., Hadgraft, J. and Wilding, I. The influence of urea on percutaneous absorption. *Pharmaceutical Research*, **3**, 294–297, 1986
25. Tyle, P. Iontophoretic devices for drug delivery. *Pharmaceutical Research*, **3**, 318–326, 1986

26. Tyle, P. and Agrawala, P. Drug delivery by phonophoresis. *Pharmaceutical Research*, **6**, 355–361, 1989
27. Kari, B. Control of blood glucose levels in alloxan-diabetic rabbits by iontophoresis of insulin. *Diabetes*, **35**, 217–221, 1986
28. Lui, J-C., Sun, Y., Siddiqui, O., Chien, Y. W., Shi, W. and Li, J. Blood glucose control in diabetic rats by transdermal iontophoretic delivery of insulin. *International Journal of Pharmaceutics*, **44**, 197–204, 1988
29. Marecki, N. M. Design considerations in transdermal drug delivery systems. *Abstracts, 10th Pharmaceutical Technology Conference, East Rutherford, N.J.* pp. 311–318, 1987 (unpublished)
30. Gienger, G., Knoch, A. and Merkle, H. P. Modelling and numerical computation of drug transport in laminates: model case evaluation of transdermal delivery system. *Journal of Pharmaceutical Sciences*, **75**, 9–15, 1986
31. Pfister, W. R., Sheeran, M. A., Watters, D. E., Sweet, R. P. and Walters, P. A. Methods for altering release of progesterone, testosterone, propranolol, and indomethacin from silicone matrices: effects of co-solvents and inert fillers. *Abstracts, Proceedings of the 14th International Symposium on Controlled Release of Bioactive Materials, Toronto*, pp. 223–224, 1987 (unpublished)
32. Karim, A. Transdermal absorption of nitroglycerin from microseal drug delivery (MDD) system. *Angiology*, **34**, 11–22, 1983
33. Skelly, J. P., Shah, V. P., Maibach, H. I., Guy, R. H., Wester, R. C., Flynn, G. L. and Yacobi, A. FDA and AAPS report of the workshop on principles and practices of in vitro percutaneous penetration studies: relevance to bioavailability and bioequivalence. *Pharmaceutical Research*, **4**, 265–267, 1987
34. PMA Committee Report: Transdermal drug delivery systems. *Pharmacopeial Forum*, **12**, 1798–1807, 1986
35. Abrams, J. Nitrate delivery systems in perspective. A decade of progress. *American Journal of Medicine*, **76**, 38–46, 1984
36. Chu, L-C., Gale, R. M., Schmitt, L. G. and Shaw, J. E. Nitroglycerin concentration in plasma: comparison between transdermal therapeutic system and ointment. *Angiology*, **35**, 545–552, 1984
37. Powers, M. S., Schenkel, L., Darley, P. E., Good, W. R., Balestra, J. C. and Place, V. A. Pharmacokinetics and pharmacodynamics of transdermal dosage forms of 17β-estradiol: comparison with conventional oral estrogens used for hormone replacement. *American Journal of Obstetrics and Gynecology*, **152**, 1099–1106, 1985
38. Good, W. R., Powers, M. S., Campbell, P. and Schenkel, L. A new transdermal delivery system for estradiol. *Journal of Controlled Release*, **2**, 89–97, 1985
39. Shaw, J. E. Transdermal therapeutic systems. In *Dermal and Transdermal Absorption* (eds R. Brandau and B. H. Lippold), Wissenschaftliche Verlagsgesellschaft, Stuttgart, pp. 171–187, 1982
40. MacGregor, T. R., Matzek, K. M., Keirns, R. G. A., van Wayjen, R. G. A., van den Ende, A. and van Tol, R. G. L. Pharmacokinetics of transdermally delivered clonidine. *Clinical Pharmacology and Therapeutics*, **38**, 278–284, 1985
41. Vlasses, P. H., Ribeiro, L. G. T., Rotmensch, H. H., Bondi, J. V., Loper, A. E., Hichens, M., Dunlay, M. C. and Ferguson, R. K. Initial evaluation of transdermal timolol: serum concentrations and β-blockade. *Journal of Cardiovascular Pharmacology*, **7**, 245–250, 1985
42. Findlay, J. C., Place, V. A. and Snyder, P. J. Transdermal delivery of testosterone. *Journal of Clinical Endocrinology and Metabolism*, **64**, 266–268, 1987

43. Behl, C. R., Kumar, S., Malick, A. W., DelTerzo, S., Higuchi, W. I. and Nash, R. A. Iontophoretic drug delivery: effects of physicochemical factors on the skin uptake of nonpeptide drugs. *Journal of Pharmaceutical Sciences*, **78**, 355–360, 1989

Further reading

Barry, B. W. *Dermatological Formulations. Percutaneous Absorption*, Marcel Dekker, New York, 1983

Chien, Y. W. (ed.) *Transdermal Controlled Systemic Medication*, Marcel Dekker, New York, 1987

Hadgraft, J. and Guy, R. H. (eds) *Transdermal Drug Delivery*, Marcel Dekker, New York, 1989

Marzulli, F. N. and Maibach, H. I. (eds) *Dermatotoxicology*, 3rd edn, Hemisphere Publishing, Washington, 1987

Shroot, B. and Schaefer, H. (eds) *Skin Pharmacokinetics*, Karger, Basle, 1987

5
Innovative methods of antibiotic administration

L. H. Danziger and J. A. Shwed

Introduction

Generally, antibiotics are administered either orally or intra-venously in the treatment of most infections. Many of the dosage schedules and techniques of administration for various antibiotics have been established in an extremely arbitrary fashion. Questions about appropriate antibiotic use still remain to be answered: what is the dose needed; what is the proper interval between doses; what is the appropriate duration of therapy? However, a more basic question concerns the most appropriate method of administering antimicrobials to treat an infectious process.

Methods of antimicrobial therapy discussed in this chapter include continuous and intermittent infusion, endotracheal installation, aerosol delivery, antibiotic-impregnated catheters, antibiotic-containing bone cement, and beads.

Continuous versus intermittent infusion

Whether antibiotics should be given by continuous infusion or by intermittent bolus injection is still controversial. Both the experimental and clinical data available concerning this question are limited, and there is a lack of evidence for superiority of either mode of administration[1, 2]. It is the general belief that adequate antimicrobial therapy requires a sustained serum concentration above the minimum inhibitory concentration (MIC) for a particular organism in the blood[1]: what is not known is for how long the concentration must be above the MIC.

Intermittent dosing is generally defined as the administration of antibiotics following a schedule which results in the serum concentration of drug falling at regular intervals below the MIC for the microorganism. The goal of continuous therapy is to maintain the serum concentration of the antibiotic above the MIC for a given microorganism at all times throughout the dosing interval.

Another consideration of equal importance to the effect of the dose interval on efficacy is its potential for toxicity. Besides understanding the pharmacokinetics of tissue penetration of antimicrobial agents to aid in appropriate dosing, pharmacodynamic properties such as post-antibiotic effect (PAE) and post-antibiotic leucocyte effect (PALE) are of importance in understanding how best to dose antimicrobial agents.

Research done in the 1940s and early 1950s showed that in some instances the concentration of an antibiotic in the serum need not exceed the MIC of the organism continuously to be effective. This concept of PAE was primarily worked out by Eagle and colleagues[3], who indicated that successful therapy depended upon the magnitude and timing of the doses used. Their research evaluated penicillin in the treatment of streptococcal infections in mice: using doses of penicillin ranging from 0.2 to 0.8 mg/kg they found 'safe' periods for only 3–6 h, whereas 'safe' periods lasted for 12–24 h when a dose of 50 mg/kg was used. They noted that this effect was found at similar concentrations both *in vitro* and *in vivo*.

Bundtzen *et al.* [4] more recently evaluated the PAE on both Gram-positive and Gram-negative bacteria *in vitro*. Although these investigators noted a PAE for all drugs studied, there were marked differences both between antibiotics and between microorganisms.

The duration of PAEs and the drug concentrations required to produce them varied for the different bacterial species. For the β-lactam antibiotics, PAEs of 1–3 h duration were noted when tested against Gram-positive organisms. However, with Gram-negative microorganisms many of these antibiotics failed to show a PAE even at four times the MIC. In general, to produce a PAE against Gram-negative bacteria much higher concentrations of the β-lactam antibiotics were required, and recovery of the bacteria was much quicker, compared with that of Gram-positive bacteria.

Post-antibiotic leucocyte effect (PALE) is a somewhat related phenomenon. McDonald and coworkers[5] found that enhanced phagocytosis and intracellular killing occurred after exposure of bacteria to certain antibiotics. These researchers speculated that the PALE operated through some increased susceptibility of antibiotic-damaged bacteria to the killing action of leucocytes.

These observations of PAE and PALE may help to explain the reported efficacy of antimicrobial regimens in which drug levels fall below the MIC for some portion of the dosing interval.

Gerber et al. [6] studied neutropenic mice infected with Pseudomonas aeruginosa. These animals were given injections of ticarcillin, gentamicin, or both, every hour or every 3 h. The results showed that the gentamicin injected every hour tended to be less active than the gentamicin given every 3 h; in contrast, ticarcillin given every hour was significantly more efficacious than the equivalent dose given every 3 h. Robinson [7], utilizing a mouse thigh model, demonstrated that when serum drug concentrations were maintained above the MIC, fewer Ps. aeruginosa cells were present at the site of infection than when the serum concentrations were allowed to fall below the MIC. Sande et al. [8] evaluated a model for continuous versus intermittent therapy with penicillin G in the treatment of Streptococcus pneumoniae meningitis in rabbits. Intermittent therapy achieved higher peaks and lower trough concentrations in the cerebrospinal fluid of the test animals. Although the initial bactericidal rate was greater in the intermittent group, after the second hour the rate of bacterial killing was identical in both groups. More recently, Thauvin et al. [9] evaluated continuous infusion ampicillin and the same total dose administered intermittently (given in three divided doses intramuscularly) for the treatment of Streptococcus faecalis endocarditis (rat model). The ampicillin infusion was found to increase the survival of the animals significantly, as well as the number of sterile blood cultures; a significant reduction in bacterial titres within the cardiac tissues was also reported for the continuous infusion therapy.

In humans, some studies evaluating continuous and intermittent dosing regimens have been done, but mostly in granulocytopenic patients receiving aminoglycosides [2, 10, 11]. Overall, these studies have not reported any differences in efficacy or toxicity. However, in the study by Bodey and coworkers [10], a subset of patients who had bacteraemia caused by a single Gram-negative bacillus responded better to continuous administration of β-lactam antibiotics, with a significant difference in positive outcomes (74% for continuous administration versus 59% for intermittent therapy). Furthermore, for those patients who had neutrophil counts of $<100/mm^3$ initially and throughout the course of the infection, the continuous administration of a β-lactam antibiotic was significantly more efficacious than intermittent therapy (65% versus 21%). Daenen and

De Vries-Hospers [12] successfully used continuous infusions of ceftazidime to treat pseudomonal skin lesions in two patients who were granulocytopenic. Both had previously been receiving intermittent ceftazidime, 2 g every 8 h, for 5–7 days without improvement, but following administration of a 2 g loading dose and a 250 mg/h continuous infusion both patients responded rapidly. Colding and coworkers [13] administered continuously, via parenteral nutrition solutions, ampicillin and gentamicin to 36 newborns with suspected septicaemia. Doses of these agents were selected to maintain a serum concentration of 40 and 4 µg/ml for ampicillin and gentamicin respectively. Utilizing continuous infusion therapy, these researchers reported outcomes equivalent to those seen with intermittent therapy.

Some other research supports the use of continuous administration of antibiotics for more satisfactory results. Anderson, Young and Hewitt [14] observed septic breakthroughs (documented by positive blood cultures) during intermittent antibiotic therapy in 12 of 19 patients when serum antibiotic concentrations fell below the MIC for the microorganism being treated.

In trying to determine whether the most appropriate dosing regimen is intermittent or continuous, the type of infection, the causative microorganism, the immunological status of the patient and the antimicrobial agent must be considered. Certain types of infection, depending on the causative microorganism, may be best treated by one rather than the other method. Limited data support the concept of high intermittent doses in the treatment of meningitis, endocarditis and Gram-negative bronchopneumonias [6, 18, 15]. In the treatment of neutropenic patients, β-lactam antibiotics may be most effective when given continuously for bacteraemias caused by Gram-negative bacilli [10,12].

Endotracheal or aerosolized instillation of antimicrobials

Hospital-acquired Gram-negative pneumonias occur in approximately 10–15% of all patients in intensive care settings. Gram-negative bronchopneumonias (GNBP) are among the most dangerous of nosocomial infections: despite recent advances in antibiotic therapy and respiratory care, the prognosis remains poor, with mortality figures ranging from 50 to 70% [16]. Patients who have depressed levels of consciousness or reflexes, or those on mechanical ventilation who develop atelectasis, are predisposed to the development of broncho-pneumonia. These pulmonary infections are usually caused by Gram-negative organisms, most commonly *Pseudomonas aerugi-nosa*[16]; unfortunately, GNBP caused by *Pseudomonas* species are the most resistant to standard antimicrobial therapy.

The reasons for poor results in the treatment of GNBP with standard antibiotic therapy have been investigated. Aminogly-cosides, the mainstay of antibiotic therapy for GNBP, penetrate rather poorly through the 'blood–bronchus barrier' after systemic administration[17, 18] and therefore sputum concen-trations above the MIC for certain microorganisms are often not achieved, despite adequate serum levels. It has also been reported that inactivation of aminoglycosides may occur in purulent secretions, thus leading to a loss of antibiotic activity at the site of infection[19]. A correlation between the antimicrobial activity in sputum and clinical outcome in bronchopulmonary infections has been shown[20].

In an attempt to overcome the low sputum concentrations from systemically administered aminoglycosides, investigators have administered these antibiotics locally into the bronchopul-monary tree. Topical antibiotic therapy may be accomplished by either of two methods: aerosolization utilizing respiratory equipment, or direct instillation endotracheally. The relative merits of these two techniques are not entirely clear. Studies conducted in animals and humans indicate that both techniques result in high and sustained aminoglycoside concentrations in bronchial secretions[21, 22]. However, some data suggest that aerosolization does not evenly distribute antibiotic to distal portions of the bronchial tree, and a recent review of the clinical data showed that the evidence for the efficacy of this method was weak[23, 24].

A theoretical advantage of endotracheally administered aminoglycosides is that with local delivery of the drug there is little or no risk of the toxicity sometimes associated with systemic administration. However, Crosby et al.[25] reported systemic absorption of from 1.5 to 34% (mean 16.7 ± 11.4%) of the total dose of aminoglycosides administered endotracheally: therefore, in some patients, e.g. those with impaired renal function, concern for toxicity attributable to systemic absorption is warranted. Endotracheally administered aminoglycosides have been shown to be effective in reducing colonization of the respiratory tract by potentially pathogenic organisms. The treatment of established GNBP with endotracheally administered aminoglycosides, on the other hand, has not yet been thoroughly investigated.

Uncontrolled studies of aminoglycosides given endotracheally[26] or by aerosol[27] have been reported to be successful. Recently, Sorenson and coworkers[28] reported a favourable response in five patients with Gram-negative pneumonia when endotracheally administered aminoglycosides were used in addition to systemic therapy; only after initiation of endotracheal gentamicin/tobramycin (40 mg every 4 h), or amikacin (200 mg every 4 h), was clinical and bacteriological improvement noted.

The best-controlled studies have been done with the aminoglycoside sisomicin administered endotracheally. Klastersky and associates[29] investigated the use of endotracheally administered sisomicin in the treatment of GNBP. Two treatment groups were compared: one received systemic sisomicin and carbenicillin plus endotracheal sisomicin; the other received only systemic carbenicillin and sisomicin. The investigators reported a favourable response in 77% of patients receiving antibiotics both parenterally and endotracheally, compared with 45% of patients receiving only parenteral antibiotics.

In a more recent randomized study, the same investigators[30] studied neurosurgical patients with GNBP: 10 patients received systemic mezlocillin plus endotracheal sisomicin; 10 other patients were randomized to receive systemic sisomicin and mezlocillin plus endotracheally administered sisomicin. Both groups were treated for slightly over one week and had similar response rates (70% for systemic mezlocillin plus endotracheal sisomicin versus 60% for systemic mezlocillin and sisomicin plus sisomicin endotracheally). In this study, systemic antibiotics were of little benefit in the treatment of GNBP.

During the past decade, aerosolized aminoglycosides and antipseudomonal penicillins have been administered to patients with cystic fibrosis for treatment of chronic bronchopulmonary pneumonia, the goals of therapy being to reduce acute attacks by suppressing colonization and to treat acute episodes of pneumonia effectively. However, often the results of clinical trials have been contradictory and inconclusive[31]. Stead and coworkers[32] recently compared ceftazidime with carbenicillin, gentamicin and placebo in a blind crossover study, with administration by nebulization. Patients experienced clinically significant improvements in indices of pulmonary function (forced expiratory volume in 1 s, forced vital capacity and peak expiratory flow), with a significant reduction in the number of hospitalizations for acute attacks of pneumonia. Other investigators have documented similar results when treating patients with cystic fibrosis colonized with *Pseudomonas aeruginosa* [33, 34]. However, conclusive evidence of the long-term benefits of aerosolized antibiotic administration in patients with cystic fibrosis is lacking. Well-controlled trials of duration ≥1 year are required, to adequately evaluate effects on morbidity and, more specifically, any progressive decline in pulmonary function.

Animal and human data have recently been reported evaluating the use of aerosolized pentamidine for the treatment or prophylaxis of *Pneumocystis carinii* pneumonia (PCP) [35, 36]. These initial reports suggested that aerosol administration of pentamidine is as effective as, and less toxic than, systemic administration in the treatment of PCP. Montgomery *et al.* [37] noted substantial objective and subjective improvement in patients receiving aerosolized pentamidine (300 mg daily for 21 days) for primary episodes of PCP; side-effects were minimal and consisted primarily of bronchospasm. More recently, Montgomery *et al.* [38] documented the improvement after aerosolized pentamidine in ten patients who had developed serious adverse effects on conventional treatment. Clinical trials have not yet been conducted to study the efficacy of aerosolized pentamidine in patients with severe disease or those who are deteriorating while on conventional therapy. Aerosolized pentamidine has also been evaluated in prophylaxis of PCP. Preliminary reports indicate that doses of 300 mg once every 2 weeks, or 2 mg/kg every 2 weeks, or 60 mg every week for 4 weeks and then bi-weekly, reduce the incidence of relapse [39, 40]. Further prospective comparative trials are needed to determine frequency, duration and doses for effective prophylaxis.

It is likely that patients without any underlying lung disease, or predisposing factors that decrease pulmonary clearance of bacteria, or underlying immune deficiency, would not benefit from the local instillation of antibiotics. In these patients the normal host defence mechanisms are adequate for fighting and/or preventing pulmonary infections. However, when patients have a damaged or impaired pulmonary system, the experimental and limited clinical data available support the local instillation of antibiotics into the bronchopulmonary system in the treatment of GNBP, and possibly the use of aerosolized pentamidine in the treatment or prevention of *Pneumocystis carinii* pneumonia.

Antibiotic-impregnated catheters

Both temporary and permenently implanted catheters are very often the starting point of hospital-acquired infections. Gram-positive bacteria, especially staphylococci, are the most frequent cause of such catheter-related infections, for reasons that are not yet clear. The antimicrobial therapies used to treat these infections are frequently inadequate and often the implicated catheter must be removed.

Peters and associates[41] noted some interesting features of bacteria–catheter interactions. They examined different catheters made of polyethylene, polyvinylchloride, polyester-based polymer, or fluorine-impregnated materials. The catheters were incubated in a nutrient-free phosphate buffer solution with coagulase-negative staphylococci, the growth of which was followed by scanning electron microscopy. Over a 96 h period, in addition to the adherence of staphylococci to both the exterior and interior surfaces of the catheter, possible breakdown of the catheter components and production of a 'slimy' material covering the bacterial colonies was noted. Apparently, bacteria (and staphylococci in particular) can grow on the catheter itself and produce a potentially protective substance that might interfere with the action of antibiotics used in treating the infection. The potential benefit of impregnating catheters with antibiotics has therefore been examined.

Trooskin and coworkers[42] evaluated the use of a silastic catheter bonded to, or soaked with, penicillin in rats undergoing simulated chronic ambulatory peritoneal dialysis. Catheters that were either bonded to (using the surfactant tridodecylmethyl-ammonium chloride, TDMAC), or soaked with, penicillin were injected with 10^3–10^{10} *Staphylococcus aureus* organisms. Both forms of penicillin-impregnated catheter significantly ($P < 0.05$) increased the dose of bacteria required to produce infection in 50% of rats: catheters with bonded antibiotic required 10^9 bacteria and soaked catheters $10^{7.7}$ organisms, compared with $10^{3.4}$ staphylococci for tubes soaked in plain TDMAC. Approximately 25% of the penicillin was still present on the TDMAC–penicillin catheter after 3 months.

The efficacy of an aminoglycoside (dibekacin sulphate)-coated in-dwelling urinary catheter was recently reported[43]. Silicone urethral catheters with ionically bonded dibekacin released aminoglycoside in concentrations above the MIC for many urinary tract pathogens. Patients with these catheters in place were found to have sterile urine for up to 8 days; however, the condition of patients with bacteriuria was not improved by these catheters.

Recently, silver ions have been evaluated for prevention of infection associated with central venous catheters and urinary drainage systems. Schaeffer and coworkers[44] investigated a catheter system which included a silver oxide-coated silicone urethral catheter, a silver oxide adapter and 20 g trichloroisocy-anuric acid added to the drainage bag to prevent bacteriuria. The incidence of bacteriuria was reduced to 29% in the treatment group versus 55% in the control group, and the onset was also significantly delayed in the treatment group (median 36 days, control group median 8 days).

Silver-impregnated catheter cuffs have been evaluated for the prevention of septicaemia and local site infections associated with central venous catheters. These infections are most often related to invasion by the patient's own skin flora[45]. Maki *et al.*[46] prospectively evaluated cuffs made with biodegradable collagen impregnated with silver and attached to Hickmann or Broviac catheters; the cuff acted as both a mechanical and a chemical barrier to microorganisms. Local catheter infections occurred in 28.9% of patients in the control group and 9.1% of patients in the silver-treated catheter group ($P=0.002$). Septicaemia occurred in 3.7% and 1% of the control and silver-treated cuff groups respectively ($P=0.12$). Differences in infection rates became more apparent, the longer the catheters were in place.

Considering the difficulties in treating catheter-related infections with systemic antibiotic therapy (the failure of which necessitates withdrawal of the tube), antibiotic-bonded or silver-impregnated catheters may be a prophylactic alternative; more research in this area is needed.

Antibiotic-impregnated bone cement

Deep bone infections are a serious complication of hip-joint replacement surgery. The routine use of systemic antibiotics for prophylaxis against infection during this type of surgery has reduced postoperative deep bone infections to the 1–2% range. In 1970 Buchholz and Engelbrecht suggested that the incorporation of an antibiotic (in this case gentamicin) in the bone cement might be a useful technique for prophylaxis of postoperative infections in orthopaedic surgery[47]. Bone cement consists of two components which, upon mixing, polymerize and harden within minutes. Theoretically, a suitable antibiotic for use in an acrylic bone cement should be water soluble, stable at body temperature and be able to resist degradation by the extreme temperatures (up to 100°C) produced during the exothermic reaction that occurs upon mixing the two components of the cement.

Marks and associates[48] studied the problems of antibiotic degradation and antibiotic diffusion out of bone cement in a dog model. They studied two types of bone cement, Simplex and Palacos, with oxacillin, cefazolin or gentamicin incorporated into them. The antibiotics (as powders) were stable in the cements; they had no influence upon compressive and diametral tension strengths of the cements, and high bactericidal concentrations were measured for *Staphylococcus aureus*, *Escherichia coli*, and *Pseudomonas aeruginosa* in surrounding bone up to 21 days after implantation. It was also noted that greater amounts of antibiotics were released from the Palacos cement than from the Simplex cement, and for longer periods.

The data available for evaluation of prospective trials comparing bone cement with other treatments in humans are scant. Petty and coworkers[49] compared polymethylmethacrylate (PMMA)-gentamicin bone cement with placebo, saline or neomycin irrigation and systemic cephazolin, in a canine model for total joint replacement. All animals received an instillation into the operative wound site of a bacterial suspension of either *Staph. aureus*, *Staph. epidermidis*, or *E. coli*. Postoperative infection was significantly less in the PMMA-gentamicin group (no infections) compared with the other treatment groups, except for the group receiving systemic cephazolin (when infected with *Staph. epidermidis* or *E. coli*).

Josefsson and associates[50] studied >1500 patients undergoing total hip arthroplasty in a prospective randomized fashion; significantly more initial superficial infections occurred in patients receiving gentamicin-impregnated cement without systemic antibiotics, compared with systemic administration of antibiotics alone ($P < 0.05$). All infections healed without complications. Altogether, 16 deep infections were later documented, 13 (1.6%) in the systemic antibiotic group and three (0.4%) in the group receiving only gentamicin-impregnated bone cement.

In the United States the Simplex cement is used most frequently; Palacos and CMW cement are used most often in Europe. The most commonly used antibiotic in bone cement has been gentamicin sulphate; generally, 1–2 g is added to 40 g cement powder. Well over 10 000 patients in Europe have been treated with this combination after total hip arthroplasty, with only minor reports of side-effects or the development of bacterial resistance. However, many of the studies have crucial design flaws, making the data difficult to interpret.

The use of antibiotic bone cement has, until recently, been limited to prophylaxis of total joint arthroplasty. Recently Garvin and coworkers[51] described the use of antibiotic-impregnated bone cement in combination with systemic therapy during one- or two-stage revision of infected total joints. In this open trial the overall rate of recurrent infection was 3.8% at 32 months of follow-up, for both the high- and low-risk groups. High-risk patients were defined as those with clinical and systemic signs and symptoms of infection. This infection rate compares favourably with historical controls (10% infection rate is generally acceptable for this patient population). Comparative blind studies in which systemic antibiotics are administered with or without antibiotic-impregnated bone cement are needed before its benefit can be assessed in a valid manner.

As only negligible serum concentrations are found after use of aminoglycoside-impregnated bone cement, this delivery system has less potential for toxicity than systemic therapy with the same antibiotic[52]. The efficacy and low toxicity support the concept of aminoglycoside-impregnated bone cement as an effective alternative or adjunct to systemic therapy for the prophylaxis of deep bone infections after total hip arthroplasty. However, because of the differences in the release of antibiotics from Palacos and Simplex cements, and design flaws in the clinical trials, further comparative studies are required to demonstrate any clinical advantages.

Antibiotic-impregnated beads

To overcome the problems encountered with the use of antibiotic-impregnated bone cement in osteomyelitis (e.g. prevention of drainage from the infection site and technical difficulties with removal if surgical débridement were necessary), Klemm[53] developed beads made from the same materials as the bone cement. Beads composed of polymethylmethacrylate and impregnated with gentamicin are commercially available in Europe for clinical use (Septopal, Merck). These beads are commonly referred to as G-PMMA, and are available singly or in strands on surgical wire; each bead is 7 mm in diameter, weighs 220 mg and contains 4.5 mg gentamicin. The beads are used for treatment of either soft tissue or deep bone infections.

Wahlig and associates[54] examined the release *in vitro* of gentamicin from G-PMMA beads: initially, concentrations of 400 µg/ml per bead were found, falling to 30–40 µg/ml and 10 µg/ml after 20 and 40 days, respectively. The G-PMMA beads released more antibiotic than the same amount of bone cement because of the vastly increased surface area available for diffusion. Wound secretions collected for 5 days postoperatively from patients being treated for soft-tissue or deep bone infections showed that gentamicin concentrations were well above the MIC for most of the pathogens commonly involved in orthopaedic infections[54]. However, the concentrations in serum and urine were low, irrespective of the number of beads implanted.

Goodell *et al.*[55] manufactured tobramycin–PMMA beads (3.6 mg tobramycin per bead) and evaluated them both *in vitro* and *in vivo*. Eighteen hours after implantation, wound drainage fluid contained 56.1 µg/ml tobramycin, whereas the serum concentration 15 h after implantation was 0.5 µg/ml and rose, 21 days after implantation, to 1.1 µg/ml.

Use of antibiotic-impregnated beads in the US is still limited. Recently, Scott and coworkers[56] reported the use of tobramycin- and vancomycin-impregnated beads in the treatment of chronic osteomyelitis. Tobramycin 1.2 g and/or vancomycin 1 g were added to 20 g PMMA bone cement and manufactured into beads, which were placed at the site of the chronic infection in three patients. Wound exudates were collected when possible and tobramycin and vancomycin concentrations measured. Tobramycin concentrations 8 h after placement were 436 and 475 mg/l, and at 24 h 94 and 192 mg/l in two patients; the third patient had concentrations of 40 mg/l and 3.2 mg/l at 6 days and 6 weeks, respectively. Vancomycin concentrations in one patient were 96 mg/l, 58 mg/l and 3 mg/l at 8 and 24 h and 12 days, respectively. All patients responded to treatment and had no recurrence at follow-up 3–3.5 years later. The authors were unable to comment on the stability or diffusion characteristics of this antibiotic–PMMA combination.

A number of other studies describing the clinical use of gentamicin-containing beads have been published. Greiber[57] has reviewed data presented in 11 European clinical trials involving >1200 patients treated with G-PMMA beads. Overall, early postoperative infection rates were reported to be *c.* 9%; furthermore, on follow-up at 1.5 years of a limited number of patients, a 7.5% recurrence rate for infections was reported. Recently, Calhoun and Mader[58] reviewed the use of antibiotic-impregnated beads in the treatment of chronic osteomyelitis and soft-tissue infections, and the prophylaxis of abdominal and head and neck operations. These authors estimated that antibiotic beads have a success rate of between 72 and 90% in chronic osteomyelitis, and in a limited number of trials have proved to be successful in prophylaxis of head and neck surgery and the treatment of soft-tissue infections. On the other hand, PMMA–gentamicin beads placed intraperitoneally for prophylaxis in colorectal surgery have not been beneficial, even when used in conjunction with systemic antibiotics. Their use was discouraged because of the development of resistant microorganisms and the pain associated with the removal of the beads.

The data available from the European studies indicate that the use of G-PMMA beads, together with débridement, may be an alternative to standard modes of therapy for osteomyelitis. However, further work with well-controlled studies is required to establish their usefulness. For use as a prophylactic regimen, however, the data available are still too limited to draw any firm conclusions about efficacy. Overall, the major obstacles to the use of antibiotic-impregnated beads are the potential for antimicrobial resistance, pain upon removal of beads (in some instances requiring general anaesthesia) and the risk of losing beads within the implantation site (which may require surgery for removal).

Conclusion

The goal of antibiotic therapy is either to cure some underlying infectious process or to prevent development of an infection. Two factors sometimes hinder the accomplishment of these goals by systemic administration of antimicrobial agents: their toxicity, or failure to reach the site of infection. Innovative and unique methods of drug administration, such as those discussed in this chapter, can often overcome these obstacles.

References

1. Eagle, H., Fleischman, R. and Levy, M. Continuous vs discontinuous therapy with penicillin. The effect of the interval between injections on therapeutic efficacy. *New England Journal of Medicine*, **248**, 481–488, 1953

2. Feld, R., Valdivieso, M., Bodey, G. P. and Rodriguez, V. A comparative trial of sisomicin therapy by intermittent versus continuous infusion. *American Journal of Medical Sciences*, **274**, 179–188, 1977
3. Eagle, H. and Musselman, A. D. The slow recovery of bacteria from the toxic effects of penicillin. *Journal of Bacteriology*, **58**, 475–490, 1949
4. Bundtzen, R. W., Gerber, A. U., Cohn, D. L. and Craig, W. A. Postantibiotic suppression of bacterial growth. *Reviews of Infectious Diseases*, **3**, 28–37, 1981
5. McDonald, P. J., Wetherall, B. L. and Pruul, H. Postantibiotic leukocyte enhancement: increased susceptibility of bacteria pretreated with antibiotic to the activity of leukocytes. *Reviews of Infectious Diseases*, **3**, 38–44, 1981
6. Gerber, A. U., Craig, W. A., Brugger, H.-P., Feller, C., Vastola, A. P. and Brandel, J. Impact of dosing intervals on activity of gentamicin and ticarcillin against *Pseudomonas aeruginosa* in granulocytopenic mice. *Journal of Infectious Diseases*, **147**, 910–917, 1983
7. Robinson, G. Basis and results of therapy with beta-lactam antibiotics in experimental infections. *Infection*, **8** (Suppl.), S30–S34, 1980
8. Sande, M. A., Korzeniowski, O. M., Allegro, G. M., Brennan, R. O., Zak, O. and Scheld, W. M. Intermittent or continuous therapy of experimental meningitis due to *Streptococcus pneumoniae* in rabbits. *Reviews of Infectious Diseases*, **3**, 98–110, 1981
9. Thauvin, C., Eliopoulos, G. M., Willey, S., Wennersten, C. and Moellering, R. C., Jr. Continuous-infusion ampicillin therapy of enterococcal endocarditis in rats. *Antimicrobial Agents and Chemotherapy*, **31**, 139–143, 1987
10. Bodey, G., Ketchel, S. and Rodriguez, V. A randomized study of carbenicillin plus cefamandole or tobramycin in the treatment of febrile episodes in cancer patients. *American Journal of Medicine*, **67**, 608–616, 1979
11. Bodey, G. P., Rodriguez, V., Valdivieso, M. and Feld, R. Amikacin for treatment of infections in patients with malignant diseases. *Journal of Infectious Diseases*, **134** (Suppl.), S421–S427, 1976
12. Daenen, S. and De Vries-Hospers, H. Cure of *Pseudomonas aeruginosa* infection in neutropenic patients by continuous infusion of ceftazidime. *Lancet*, **i**, 937, 1988
13. Colding, H., Moller, S. and Andersen, G. Continuous intravenous infusion of ampicillin and gentamicin during parenteral nutrition to 36 newborn infants using a dosage schedule. *Acta paediatrica scandinavica*, **73**, 203–209, 1984
14. Anderson, E., Young, L. and Hewitt, W. Simultaneous antibiotic levels in 'breakthrough' Gram-negative bacteremia. *American Journal of Medicine*, **61**, 493–497, 1976
15. Klastersky, J., Thys, J. P. and Mombelli, G. Comparative studies of intermittent and continuous administration of aminoglycosides in the treatment of bronchopulmonary infections due to Gram-negative bacteria. *Reviews of Infectious Diseases*, **3**, 74–83, 1981
16. Stevens, R. M., Teres, D., Skillman, J. J. and Feingold, D. S. Pneumonia in the intensive care unit. *Archives of Internal Medicine*, **134**, 106–111, 1974
17. Pennington, J. E. Penetration of antibiotics into respiratory secretions. *Reviews of Infectious Diseases*, **3**, 67–73, 1981
18. Alexander, M. The concentrations of tobramycin in bronchial secretions. *Chest*, **75**, 675–681, 1979
19. Bryant, R. Interactions of purulent material with antibiotics used to treat pseudomonal infections. *Antimicrobial Agents and Chemotherapy*, **6**, 702–704, 1974
20. May, J. and Delves, D. Treatment of chronic bronchitis with ampicillin. *Lancet*, **i**, 929–933, 1965

21. Braun, J., Kundren, D. and Sorekin, S. Pulmonary distribution of particles by endotracheal administration or by aerosol inhalation. *Environmental Research*, **11**, 13–33, 1976
22. Ramirez, J. and O'Neill, R. A. Endotracheal polymyxin B. *Chest*, **58**, 352–357, 1970
23. Patterson, C. and Kamp, G. Retention of aerosol liquids in the lung. *American Journal of Respiratory Disease*, **95**, 443–446, 1967
24. Gough, P. and Jordan, N. A review of the therapeutic efficacy of aerosolized and endotracheally instilled antibiotics. *Pharmacotherapy*, **2**, 367–377, 1982
25. Crosby, S. S., Edwards, W. A. D., Brennan, C., Dellinger, E. P. and Bauer, L. A. Systemic absorption of endotracheally administered aminoglycosides in seriously ill patients with pneumonia. *Antimicrobial Agents and Chemotherapy*, **31**, 850–853, 1987
26. Bibodean, M., Ray, J. and Grioux, M. Studies of absorption of kanamycin by aerosolization. *Annals of the New York Academy of Sciences*, **132**, 870–878, 1966
27. Klastersky, J., Geuning, C. and Mouawad, E. Endotracheal gentamicin in bronchial infections in patients with tracheostomy. *Chest*, **61**, 117–120, 1972
28. Sorenson, V. J., Horst, H. M. and Obeid, F. N. Endotracheal aminoglycosides in Gram-negative pneumonia. *American Surgeon*, **52**, 391–394, 1986
29. Klastersky, J., Carpentier-Meunier, F., Kahan-Coppens, L. and Thys, J. P. Endotracheally administered antibiotics for Gram-negative bronchopneumonia. *Chest*, **75**, 586–591, 1971
30. Sculier, J. P., Coppens, L. and Klastersky, J. Effectiveness of mezlocillin and endotracheally administered sisomicin with or without parenteral sisomicin in the treatment of Gram-negative bronchopneumonia. *Journal of Antimicrobial Chemotherapy*, **9**, 63–68, 1982
31. MacLusky, I., Levison, H., Gold, R. and McLaughlin, F. J. Inhaled antibiotics in cystic fibrosis: is there a therapeutic effect? *Journal of Pediatrics*, **108**, 861–865, 1986
32. Stead, R. J., Hodson, M. E. and Batten, J. C. Inhaled ceftazidime compared with gentamicin and carbenicillin in older patients with cystic fibrosis infected with *Pseudomonas aeruginosa*. *British Journal of Diseases of the Chest*, **81**, 272–279, 1987
33. Carswell, F., Ward, C., Cook, D. A. and Speller, D. C. E. A controlled trial of nebulized aminoglycoside and oral flucloxacillin versus placebo in the outpatient management of children with cystic fibrosis. *British Journal of Diseases of the Chest*, **81**, 356–360, 1987
34. Hodson, M. E. Antibiotic treatment: aerosol therapy. *Chest*, **94** (Suppl.), 156S–160S, 1988
35. Conte, J., Hollander, H. and Golden, J. Inhaled or reduced dose intravenous pentamidine for *Pneumocystis carinii* pneumonia. *Annals of Internal Medicine*, **107**, 495–498, 1987
36. Girard, P.-M., Brun-Pascaud, M., Farinotti, R., Tamisier, L. and Kernbaum, S. Pentamidine in prophylaxis and treatment of murine *Pneumocystis carinii* pneumonia. *Antimicrobial Agents and Chemotherapy*, **31**, 978–981, 1987
37. Montgomery, A. B., Debs, R. J., Luce, J. M., Corkery, K. J., Turner, J., Brunette, E. H., Lin, E. T. and Hopewell, P. C. Aerosolized pentamidine as sole therapy for *Pneumocystis carinii* pneumonia in patients with acquired immuno-deficiency syndrome. *Lancet*, ii, 480–483, 1987
38. Montgomery, A. B., Debs, R. J., Luce, J. M., Corkery, K. J., Turner, J. and Hopewell, P. C. Aerosolized pentamidine as second line therapy in patients with AIDS and *Pneumocystis carinii* pneumonia. *Chest*, **95**, 747–750, 1989

39. Fallat, R. J., Kandal, K. and Feigal, D. Pentamidine aerosol (PA) to prevent pneumocystis pneumonia (PCP). *American Review of Respiratory Disease*, **137** (Suppl.), 120, 1988 (Abstract)
40. Van Gundy, K. P., Akil, B., Bill, R. and Boylen, C. T. The effect of inhaled pentamidine on prevention of *Pneumocystis carinii* pneumonia in patients with acquired immuno-deficiency syndrome (AIDS). *American Review of Respiratory Disease*, **137** (Suppl.), 120, 1988 (Abstract)
41. Peters, G., Locci, R. and Pulverer, G. Adherence and growth of coagulase-negative staphylococci on surfaces of intravenous catheters. *Journal of Infectious Diseases*, **146**, 479–482, 1982
42. Trooskin, S., Harvey, R. and Donely, S. Antibiotic bonded chronic peritoneal dialysis catheter. *European Journal of Surgical Research*, **17** (Suppl.), 2–3, 1985
43. Sakamoto, I., Umemura, Y. and Nakano, H. Efficacy of an antibiotic-coated indwelling catheter: a preliminary report. *Journal of Biomedical Materials Research*, **19**, 1031–1041, 1985
44. Schaeffer, A. J., Story, K. O. and Johnson, S. M. Effect of silver oxide/trichloroisocyanuric acid antimicrobial urinary drainage system on catheter associated bacteriuria. *Journal of Urology*, **139**, 69–73, 1988
45. Maki, D. and Ringer, M. Evaluation of dressing regimens for prevention of infection with peripheral intravenous catheters. *Journal of the American Medical Association*, **258**, 2396–2403, 1987
46. Maki, D. G., Cobb, L., Garman, J. K., Shapiro, J. M., Ringer, M. and Helgerson, R. B. An attachable silver-impregnated cuff for prevention of infection with central venous catheters: a prospective randomized multicenter trial. *American Journal of Medicine*, **85**, 307–314, 1988
47. Buchholz, H. W. and Engelbrecht, H. Über die Depotwirkung einiger Antibiotica bei Vermischung mit dem Kunstharz Palacos. *Chirurg*, **41**, 511–515, 1970
48. Marks, K. E., Nelson, C. L. and Lautenschlager, E. P. Antibiotic-impregnated acrylic bone cement. *Journal of Bone and Joint Surgery*, **58A**, 358–359, 1976
49. Petty, W., Spanier, S. and Shuster, J. J. Prevention of infections after total joint replacement: experiments with a canine model. *Journal of Bone and Joint Surgery*, **70A**, 536–539, 1988
50. Josefsson, G., Lindberg, L. and Wiklander, B. Systemic antibiotics and gentamicin containing bone cement in the prophylaxis of postoperative infections in total hip arthroplasty. *Clinical Orthopedics and Related Research*, **159**, 194–200, 1981
51. Garvin, K. L., Salvati, E. A. and Brause, B. D. Role of gentamicin-impregnated cement in total joint arthroplasty. *Orthopedic Clinics of North America*, **19**, 605–610, 1988
52. Marr, M. and Alozozzine, G. Use of tobramycin bone cement. *Clinical Pharmacy*, **2**, 401, 1983
53. Klemm, K. Treatment of chronic bone infections with gentamicin PMMA chains and beads. *Accidental Surgery*, **1**, 20, 1976
54. Wahlig, H., Dingeldein, E., Bergmann, R. and Reuss, K. The release of gentamicin from polymethylmethacrylate beads. *Journal of Bone and Joint Surgery*, **60B**, 270–275, 1978
55. Goodell, J. A., Flick, A. B., Hebert, J. C. and Howe, J. G. Preparation and release characteristics of tobramycin-impregnated polymethylmethacrylate beads. *American Journal of Hospital Pharmacy*, **43**, 1454–1461, 1986

56. Scott, D. M., Rotschafer, J. C. and Behrens, F. Use of vancomycin and tobramycin polymethylmethacrylate impregnated beads in the management of chronic osteomyelitis. *Drug Intelligence and Clinical Pharmacy*, **22**, 480–483, 1988
57. Greiber, A. Treatment of bone and soft tissue infections with gentamicin polymethylmethacrylate chains. *South African Journal of Medicine*, **60**, 395–397, 1981
58. Calhoun, J. H. and Mader, J. T. Antibiotic beads in the management of surgical infections. *American Journal of Surgery*, **157**, 443–449, 1989

Index